D0193349

CHICKEN SOUP FOR THE DIETER'S SOUL

CHICKEN SOUP
FOR THE
DIETER'S SOUL

Inspiration and Humor to
Get You Over the Hump

Jack Canfield
Mark Victor Hansen
Theresa Peluso

Health Communications, Inc.
Deerfield Beach, Florida

www.hcibooks.com
www.chickensoup.com

We would like to acknowledge the many publishers and individuals who granted us permission to reprint the cited material. (Note: The stories that were penned anonymously, that are in the public domain, or that were written by Jack Canfield, Mark Victor Hansen or Theresa Peluso are not included in this listing.)

My Weight-Loss Journey. Reprinted by permission of Julia Havey. ©2005 Julia Havey.

Phone Friend. Reprinted by permission of Peggy Frezon. ©2006 Peggy Frezon.

The Swimming Lesson. Reprinted by permission of Susan Farr-Fahncke. ©2000 Susan Farr-Fahncke.

Weighing Heavily on His Mind. Reprinted by permission of Kathe M. Campbell. ©2006 Kathe M. Campbell.

Diner's Club. Reprinted by permission of Tricia Finch. ©2006 Tricia Finch.

Sit-Ups Till Your Eyes Pop Out. Reprinted by permission of Samantha Hoffman. ©2006 Samantha Hoffman.

(Continued on page 255)

Library of Congress Cataloging-in-Publication Data

Chicken soup for the dieter's soul : inspiration and humor to get you over the hump / [compiled by] Jack Canfield, Mark Victor Hansen, Theresa Peluso.
    p. cm.
  ISBN-13: 978-0-7573-0555-9 (trade paper)
  ISBN-10: 0-7573-0555-5 (trade paper)
  1. Weight loss. 2. Weight loss—Anecdotes. I. Canfield, Jack, 1944- II. Hansen, Mark Victor. III. Peluso, Theresa.
  RM222.2.C478 2007
  613.2′5—dc22

           2006033439

©2006 Jack Canfield and Mark Victor Hansen

All rights reserved. Printed in the United States of America. No part of this publication may be reproduced, stored in a retrieval system, or transmitted in any form or by any means, electronic, mechanical, photocopying, recording or otherwise without the written permission of the publisher.

HCI, its logos and marks are trademarks of Health Communications, Inc.

Publisher: Health Communications, Inc.
         3201 S.W. 15th Street
         Deerfield Beach, FL 33442–8190

Cover design by Andrea Perrine Brower
Inside book formatting by Theresa Peluso and Dawn Von Strolley Grove

We dedicate this book to
those who face the daily
challenges of
overweight and obesity.

Contents

2. EATING WELL AND STAYING FIT

3. NO PAIN . . . NO GAIN

4. INSIGHTS AND REVELATIONS

5. THE NEW YOU

Acknowledgments

Compiling, editing and publishing a book requires the energy and expertise of many people, but it begins with the support of our families, who are a perpetual source of joy and love. Thank you, Inga, Christopher, Travis, Riley, Oran, Kyle, Patty, Elisabeth, Melanie and Brian.

Behind the scenes there are dozens of talented, enthusiastic staff members, freelancers and interns who keep the wheels turning smoothly at Chicken Soup for the Soul Enterprises, Self-Esteem Seminars, Mark Victor Hansen and Associates, and Health Communications, Inc.

The vision and commitment of our publisher, Peter Vegso, brings *Chicken Soup for the Soul* to the world.

Patty Aubery and Russ Kalmaski share this journey with love, laughter and endless creativity.

Patty Hansen has handled the legal and licensing aspects of each book thoroughly and competently, and Laurie Hartman has been a precious guardian of the *Chicken Soup* brand.

Barbara LoMonaco and D'ette Corona bring their endless cooperation and incredible coordination and organization of a million details to the table, time and again.

Veronica Romero, Teresa Esparza, Robin Yerian, Jesse Ianniello, Lauren Edelstein, Jody Emme, Debbie Lefever,

Michelle Adams, Dee Dee Romanello, Shanna Vieyra, Lisa Williams, Gina Romanello, Brittany Shaw, Noelle Champagne, Tanya Jones and Mary McKay support Jack's and Mark's businesses with skill and love.

Allison Janse, our editor at Health Communications, Inc., makes every book a joy to work on through her sense of humor and her extraordinary gift with words. The incredible creative team at Health Communications— Larissa Hise-Henoch, Lawna Patterson Oldfield, Andrea Perrine Brower, Anthony Clausi, Dawn Von Strolley Grove, Bernie Herschbein and Peter Quintal—combine their gifts to make each book special.

Thank you to everyone at Health Communications, from the production team to sales, marketing, public relations and fulfillment, who get all of our books into readers' hands, copy after copy, with exacting standards and professionalism.

Readers around the world enjoy *Chicken Soup* more than thirty-six languages because of the effort of Claude Choquette and Luc Jutras at Montreal Contacts.

And our thanks and appreciation go out to Michelle Abramovitz, Jennifer Campbell, Katy McManus, Darcy Newman, Marsha and Stephan Oldfield, Victoria Patterson, Leslie Steinberner, Kim Howe, Kenneth Thompson, Andre Villanouff, and Suzanne Weaver for helping us select the best stories by generously giving their time and sharing their feedback.

To everyone who submitted a story, we deeply appreciate your letting us into your lives and sharing your experiences with us. For those whose stories were not chosen for publication, we hope the stories you are about to enjoy convey what was in your heart and in some way also tell your stories.

And last, but certainly not least, to our readers. You are the reason we strive for the best and continue to bring you the magic of *Chicken Soup for the Soul*.

Introduction

I have to confess, I'm not a dieter. I'm one of the lucky ones who got to eat anything she wanted and be relatively inactive all of my life—until I found myself a few years away from celebrating the big "50," weighing in at thirty pounds heavier and buying my third new size in jeans since my salad days. I had no stamina, energy, muscle tone or strength. My asthma and my immune system seemed to be in overdrive, making me highly reactive and allergic to dozens of things around me. Still, I couldn't bring myself to count points or calories, analyze food labels, or deny myself my comfort food.

Something had to change. For me the turning point was 9/11. After seeing so many lives senselessly wasted, I wanted to be healthy and strong—to not take the gift of life and a healthy body for granted any longer. I embraced exercise and made a commitment to eating healthier. So, although I don't consider myself a dieting veteran, I have made the journey to reclaim my health and vitality, which is what dieting is all about—or should be.

Working on this book has been an enlightening experience. Certainly, I'd heard all the news—we're fatter than ever and our children are destined for lives filled with heart disease and diabetes unless we make some major changes in our lifestyles. I knew from other work I've done that we are a culture obsessed with unattainable standards of beauty and body image issues, whether real or perceived. But I had no idea how many people suffered lifelong with their weight, dieting repeatedly, hoping for the fix (it's never quick) to be permanent (it's usually temporary.)

I sifted through hundreds of stories, and a pattern emerged. The success stories were those in which people realized their attitude had to change on a deeper level to create permanent change in their daily lives. Millions succeed to some degree or other with the popular programs and supplements that fuel a multi-billion-dollar dieting industry. But universally, more important than which program or plan dieters followed was the fact that they had finally reconciled their hearts and minds to changing their relationship to food. Success began when they chose to eat to live, not live to eat.

The "simple" truth is that we must eat a diet of nutrient-rich, balanced food groups, in smaller portions, more frequently, and we must get daily exercise. It takes effort, as you'll see from Guy Burdick's piece, "Running from a Diabetic Coma to the Marine Corps Marathon," but it can be fun, as Greg Faherty shows us in "Gone to the Dogs." Trying to go it alone can be a daunting prospect, so finding a partner or making it a family affair is a great way to stay on track. Tricia Finch learned some solid tips from her "trainer," which she shares in "Weight-Loss Wisdom from a Toddler," and Peggy Frezon dealt with her empty-nest syndrome and got some exercise at the same time in "Phone Friend."

Why we eat seems to be as important as what we eat, and we have several pieces that get to the core of the issue of emotional eating. Jacquelyn B. Fletcher shares her experiences with food and feelings in "The Road to Self-Worth," while Georgia A. Hubley's transformation described in "Monday Morning Blues" is a blueprint for dieting success.

For some, our early environment or our genes stack the odds against us. When all else fails, surgery is a viable option. Marilyn Eudaly describes how she chose gastric bypass in "The Secret." In "Whatever I Want," Perry P. Perkins tells us how growing up in poverty dictated his relationship with food. Anyone considering bariatric surgery needs to read Perry's story.

Exercise is the second, but equally essential, part of the weight management equation. Harriet Cooper met the challenge head-on and shares her insight in three pieces, "Where Money Meets Resolutions," "The Exchange Rate" and "Couch Meets Table." You may see a glimpse of yourself and have a good laugh when you read "The Exercise Bike" from Ann Morrow. And Charmi Schroeder, one of the former "stars" of a Richard Simmons's *Sweatin' to the Oldies* video, returns for an encore in an inspiring piece, "Stroke of Inspiration."

Throughout *Chicken Soup for the Dieter's Soul* you'll find delicious recipes anyone can enjoy, taken from cookbooks authored by two physicians with a special interest in diet and health. Diana Schwarzbein, a California endocrinologist and internist, developed *The Schwarzbein Principle* in the early 1990s and has since helped thousands of type 2 diabetics and insulin-resistant clients reclaim their health and take control of their well-being. Andrew Larson, a specialist in bariatric surgery, teamed up with his wife, Ivy Ingram Larson, a fitness and nutrition expert, to create a diet and exercise program after Ivy was diagnosed with multiple sclerosis in her twenties. *The Gold Coast Cure* is a life-saving program for anyone living with autoimmune or inflammatory diseases. In addition to stories, we've included a resource section to help you maximize the effectiveness of your weight-management program.

Although dieting is a solitary, personal process, we offer you *Chicken Soup for the Dieter's Soul* as a source of companionship, motivation, insight and inspiration, empathy and encouragement. And we wish you—no matter what the number on that scale may be—a healthy, strong and vibrant life, lived to the fullest.

Theresa Peluso

Share with Us

We would love to hear your reactions to the stories in this book. Please let us know what your favorite stories were and how they affected you.

We also invite you to send us stories you would like to see published in future editions of *Chicken Soup for the Soul*. You can send us either stories you have written or stories written by others. Please send submissions to:

Chicken Soup for the Soul
P.O. Box 30880
Santa Barbara, CA 93130
Fax: 805-563-2945

You can also access e-mail or find a current list of planned books at the *Chicken Soup for the Soul* website at *www.chickensoup.com*.

We hope you enjoy reading this book as much as we enjoyed compiling, editing and writing it.

1

MIND OVER MATTER

*T*his life is yours: Take the power to choose what
you want to do and do it well. Take the power
to love what you want in life and love it hon-
estly. Take the power to walk in the forest and
be a part of nature. Take the power to control
your own life. No one else can do it for you.
Take the power to make your life happy.

Susan Polis Schutz

My Weight-Loss Journey

When we move out of the familiar here and now, we set in motion a series of events that, taken together, bring about changes at the very root of our being.

Joseph Dispenza

There was a time in my life when everything was completely out of control. I was considered "morbidly obese" at 290 pounds, my marriage was horrible and I was a diet junkie but still gaining weight on every fad that I tried. Looking back, it is still difficult for me to pinpoint how I got myself into such a rut, but it is quite easy for me to explain how I broke the cycle that kept me in the downward spiral that had become my life.

At thirty years old, I felt way too young to be my mother, yet there I was, weighing 290 pounds, unhappy all the time, in debt, lonely and eating for comfort. I so desperately wanted my life to improve and laid my hopes on the belief that once I lost weight, everything would! In an attempt to solve all of my problems, I went on every popular diet that I heard about—from the cabbage soup diet to the lesser-known "cantaloupe, tuna and Diet Pepsi diet." Each diet left me overweight and disillusioned —certainly not the outcome I desired. I resigned myself to the fact that I was destined to be fat, lacked any willpower and would likely fail at any diet that I ever tried.

One day in 1994, while opening the mail, I came upon an envelope without a return address. I opened it, read it and discovered that my husband was having an affair. It was like being punched in the stomach, but the pain didn't go away. An argument ensued and I rushed out the door, needing to get away—you know, to get something to eat.

I headed to the closest gas station to buy a candy bar and there he was—the man who would facilitate my change in destiny! As I got out of my car, I gave my sweat-shirt the obligatory tug, pulling it down so that it covered my butt and thus hid my fat from the world—or so I thought. As I walked toward the attendant's window to get my food fix, this man leaning on the side of the building, drinking something out of a tattered brown paper bag and wearing clothing stained with soot and grime, loudly observed, "Girl, you got too much food in you!" Not just a quiet observation, mind you, but very loud and heckling. Repeatedly and more loudly my tormentor kept up his chanting. Everyone, even the attendant behind the bullet-proof glass window, was laughing—laughing at my fat and me. I took my candy bar and quickly retreated to my car as he got one last comment in: "Damn, girl!" I was beyond humiliated.

Enough was enough. "Too much food in me!" *I'll show him*, I thought as I sped off; giving him a parting gesture as I spun my wheels like a bat out of hell. I quickly opened up my Mounds bar and sought solace. Strangely, comfort wasn't to be found that night—not in the coconut and chocolate, not in the ice cream that I ate when I got home, and least of all, not when I took a good look in the mirror.

He was right—and it hit me hard. He hadn't meant to be cruel, but he was being honest and called it as he saw it. Sure, other people's comments could be construed as mean-spirited, but not this man's. He didn't make fun of me, he didn't call me "fat"; no, he simply stated the obvious: I had too much food in me.

I took a long look at myself and at my life that night, and I realized what the problems really were. It wasn't my husband's fault that I had gotten overweight; it wasn't my parent's fault; it wasn't the teasing; it wasn't anything that anyone else did to me—it was every bite of food that went into my mouth that didn't belong there.

From that day on, I quit thinking that simply losing weight would change me and improve my life; I realized that if I changed my actions, in time my life had no choice but to change! From that day on, I quit putting "too much food in me." It was very easy for me to identify a few foods that I had way "too much of in me"; after all, I was eating at least a half gallon of ice cream a night. That seemed like a good place to start.

My weight loss did not happen overnight and my life didn't improve overnight; but, rather, over a series of many nights, days, weeks and months I made consistent small steps in the direction of a healthier life—a well-balanced life! I literally started by changing one habit, which led to changing one more habit, and so on, which wasn't overwhelming and was very doable. I gave up my ice cream vice, "busted" fast food, started cooking and eating with my children, stopped eating in the car or in front of the TV, and started to read labels and learn about the contents of what I was consuming.

I also started getting some exercise. After I lost fifteen or twenty pounds, I joined an aerobics class. After I lost about fifty pounds, I became comfortable and more confident in myself and I started to work out more often. I began taking step classes and performing muscle-strengthening exercises. I started walking around the park with my children and playing with them in the playground.

Over the course of the next fifteen months I lost over 130 pounds—almost exactly two pounds per week—a healthy pace by all standards. My productivity at work improved, my attitude was vastly more positive and my life was finally pulling out of the downward spiral. Sadly, my marriage did not improve despite the fact that my body did. For so many years I thought that losing weight would change everything in my life and my marriage. My husband was a very nice person, but together we didn't work. Each of us had different interests and desires for our lives, and it became clear that my weight loss wasn't going to change us—*only how I looked.*

Each day is a new page in my journey, which began with a homeless man, my guardian angel, who opened my eyes, gave me a dose of reality and shocked me into changing my life. It worked!

Julia Havey

Phone Friend

The family is the essential presence—the thing that never leaves you, even if you find you have to leave it.

Bill Buford

It's too early, too cold, too hot, I'm too tired, the wind is blowing in the wrong direction . . . whatever the excuse, I'd try anything to get out of exercising! But my daughter Kate wouldn't fall for any of that. "C'mon, Mom," she'd say. "You'll feel better after you get out there and move."

Sometimes we'd go to the gym together. It was always so much easier to pound that treadmill when I saw she was sweating right beside me. Sometimes we'd play tennis. I wasn't any good, but she kept hitting those balls to me, never losing patience. And at least I'd get a lot of exercise chasing the ones that went over the fence or into the woods. "Good job," Kate would say. "Wasn't that fun?" And you know, it was when we did it together.

Last fall, though, it was time for Kate to go away to college. I was happy for her to have such an exciting opportunity, but I missed having her around. *At least now I won't have to worry about anyone dragging me out there to exercise,* I thought. But do you know what? I missed that, too.

At home, things just weren't the same. My husband worked hard at the office all day, and when he came home, he wanted to relax and unwind. The last thing he wanted to do was run off to the gym. And my fifteen-year-old son was active with soccer, basketball, and baseball practices and games. There was no one left at home to force me to push my body in ways I naturally tended to avoid.

Since I wasn't sure how to motivate myself, I ended up doing nothing. I worked from home, and pretty soon my only exercise was rolling my office chair from my desk to my computer screen and tossing wads of paper into the trash can. I did dive for the phone when it rang, though. That was when Kate would call from college.

"It's a long way to classes from my dorm," she said, "but the walking is great!" She referred to the expected weight gain for new college students. "The freshman fifteen? Not for me!"

Soon Kate called me whenever she was making that long walk to campus. She filled me in on all the exciting details of her life: inspiring courses, new friends, interesting clubs and activities. I really looked forward to her calls and connecting to her life. I cradled the phone, cozied up on the couch and settled in for a nice chat.

"You're lucky," I said one day. "I wish you were here to walk with me. You're off at school while I'm sitting here on the couch!"

"I don't think anyone's forcing you to sit around!" Kate joked.

Ouch! Of course, I knew she was right. No one was forcing me to do anything. It was a matter of choice. Maybe I just needed to choose something different.

The next day when my cell rang, I didn't plop right

down on the couch. Instead, I laced up my sneakers and headed for the front door.

"Mom, you sound a little out of breath," said Kate as we chatted. "What are you doing?"

"I'm walking, too!" I said. "I decided whenever you called, I'd get up and go around the block."

"That's great!" she replied. We talked all the way around the block three times!

Even though we were hundreds of miles apart, thanks to our cell phones we were still able to walk together. Distracted by good conversation, I didn't feel like exercise was such a task. I began to look forward to the phone ringing, reminding me to get up and move. As Kate kept fit, I did, too. And as always, the exercise felt better when we were doing it together.

Peggy Frezon

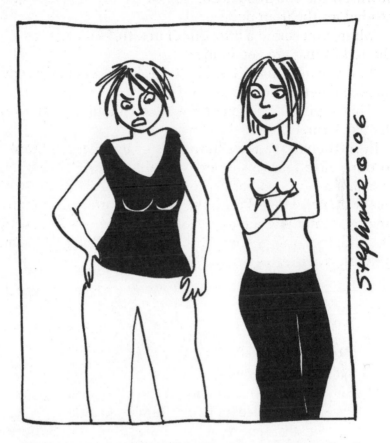

"Will you look at that! My freshman 15 has finally caught up with me . . . 20 years later!"

Reprinted with permission of Stephanie Piro.

The Swimming Lesson

*We are all dreaming of some magical rose gar-
den over the horizon—instead of enjoying the
roses that are blooming outside our windows
today.*

Dale Carnegie

Boy, did I want to swim. A water lover by nature, it was
hard for me not to dive in and let the cool water surround
me. How I love the feel of being immersed and swimming
to my heart's content. A sense of freedom and giddiness
always overcomes me when I'm half-naked in a pool.
But that was the problem. Being half-naked. After giving
birth three times, I had let myself go and the weight had
crept up on me like a thief in the night, stealing my self-
confidence and my ability to do the things I loved so
much, swimming being one of them.

Watching my family splash and laughing together in the
hotel pool was almost too much for me. I wished the other
people in the pool would disappear so I could take an
unself-conscious plunge. Glancing down at my extra-
curvy body took away what little guts I had built up.

My husband, always my greatest cheerleader, begged me to come in. "Honey, you are beautiful," he tried to reassure me. He knew why I wouldn't come in. Sitting with my Diet Coke and my baggy clothing, I shook my head and wished he'd shut up. People could hear him. I imagined they were probably thankful I wasn't donning a swimsuit.

"Please, Mom," echoed my kids, "get in!" they hollered at me. By now I was thoroughly mortified that everyone in the pool area knew I was too embarrassed to go swimming.

The blue-green water beckoned me. I thought back to the days when putting on a swimsuit was nothing more than, well, putting on a swimsuit. I would spend hours and hours playing water volleyball, laughing and racing my friends in underwater relays. I closed my eyes and could almost feel the water carry me away, freeing me from everyday life and surrounding me with good, old-fashioned fun.

I enviously watched the people in the pool, and as a few of them left, my husband tried again. "Come ON. It's no fun without you." His brown eyes almost convinced me. Almost.

He swam up to the edge of the pool, trying to persuade me. He whispered loud enough for only me to hear, "You are sexy and gorgeous to me," he reasoned. "Who else matters?"

Men are so basic. I wish I could have that thinking process.

"Mom-my, Mom-my," my kids chanted. I saw my husband whispering to each of the kids. Grinning, they all climbed out of the pool.

"We're not swimming until you get in." My husband was now using his guilt tactic—a bargaining device that is usually my expertise. I could see that he was serious, and then I realized he was right. If he wasn't embarrassed at his wife wearing a swimsuit in public, then why should I be? He knew how much I loved swimming and how hard it was for me to miss out. This was love. Real love.

The group of teenagers that I was most intimidated by finally vacated the pool. Only a few stragglers remained. I really had no excuse now. I bit my lip and involuntarily flinched at the thought of myself in a bathing suit. And yet, I knew if I missed out, I would regret it. I was tired of regretting things. I wanted for once to be glad I did something, not sorry I didn't.

Hopping up, I headed for our room and changed into my suit as quickly as I could—before I changed my mind. Beach towel wrapped around my hips, I scurried down to the pool. I flung the towel off and dove in, not a second's hesitation. When I came up for air, my family was grinning and shouting, "Go Mom!" We played for a long, long time and I loved it. I caught my husband watching me with a strange expression on his face. His eyes glimmering, he motioned me over to him. Feeling like a mermaid, I happily swam to his side.

"You are SO beautiful," he said intensely. I searched his face for some sign of embarrassment or sarcasm. All I saw was sincerity. I giggled like a sixteen-year-old and his smile grew bigger. "You should do things you like more often. You look so happy, you actually glow."

He meant it. And I vowed to never let myself stand in my way again.

Susan Farr-Fahncke

Weighing Heavily on His Mind

Flatter me, and I may not believe you. Criticize me, and I may not like you. Ignore me, and I may not forgive you. Encourage me, and I will not forget you.

William Arthur Ward

"Honey, do you think I can get into my tux?" queried my man full of wishful thoughts.

"Doubt it darlin'," I said as I gave him a pat on the mound that stood guard over his belt. My negative comment fell on deaf ears as Ken rushed to the downstairs wardrobe where his tux and my wedding dress have hung for thirty-four years. Putting on a few pounds hadn't seemed to weigh heavy on his mind despite small nags over his gluts and guzzles. Nonetheless, a wife knows when extra pounds and ill-fitting clothes bum her guy out.

Now the jig was up.

Moans and huffs spiraled up the stairs.

"This is great. The tie, cummerbund and white suspenders are still here," he hollered.

"Guess I'll have to buy a dress shirt, this one's looking pretty tired." Tugging at obstinate gaps, my darlin' emerged dressed to the nines, like Mrs. Astor's pony. He'd never be a clotheshorse with a single button threatening to take flight under sixty years of baggage. Stiff and staid and popping at the seams, he sucked in beneath an unrelenting waistband.

Bent on conquering the spare tire in days, brainstorms began spilling out. "Maybe if I went on a crash diet. I'm running into town to look at exercise machines."

Having never been faithful to our stationary bike, I questioned his motives. "Are you sure you want to torment your carcass braving the latest ab-gadgets with your arthritis? Those tummy trainers and stretch-and-roll machines look like medieval torture devices to me."

Weeks later, we made a handsome couple at the Montana Governor's Ball, despite the tuxedo fiasco. Ken was in good company, for half the men were decked out in dark suits. But journeying home, grumbles surfaced. "I felt like an old, fat man tonight! Why don't we go on one of those diets?"

We? Well yes, I could stand a belly bob and knew he'd fall off the weight wagon without a compatriot to share his misery. It would be good for our health. We did our homework, and although Ken wanted to jump in and take the first plan, we enrolled in the one best befitting our lifestyle. At weekly weigh-ins we ran into folks we had known for years, cajoling us with raves of success. The whole thing seemed so easy, and though exercise was recommended, it wasn't a prerequisite. Okay! Suddenly we were indulging in a food plan for our age group, Ken's diabetes and our doctor's hearty approval. It was as simple as adding water and nuking tasty meals three times a day. Portions and nutrition became our bible, although his majesty swore he was starving. The togetherness scheme was lobbing off unsightly bloats and pounds weekly.

Despite the taboo, we cheated on weekends, indulging in Sunday dinner out on the town. Our little gold star reward system was a comfort thing, charging diet batteries for Monday mornings. At just one hundred days, Ken's double chin and both our middles had departed into hog heaven. Forty for Ken, and my thirty-two pounds had evaporated, and we felt like a million bucks. 'Twas like being given a precious gift by someone we both loved . . . ourselves.

Now on our own, like two little kids starting first grade, that scary "maintenance" word challenged us. Snarling and goading, the new digital scale sat on the kitchen floor, underfoot in plain sight. The cat and mouse game commenced, gaining one, losing two. Our rules? Garden varieties on demand, medium-sized new and old favorites with no seconds, reasonable desserts, and no bedtime snacks. Gastronomic makeovers inside and out were leaving contented tummies and high spirits. But for good professional counseling in our economical program, we might have slid back into the potbelly pit.

The slender years rolled on and again we waited for our invitation to the governor's second-term ball. The engraved card said January 14. But this time Mr. Lean and Trim was so comfortable in his svelte person that thoughts of the old tux were ditched in lieu of more modern formal wear.

"Ya know what, hon; I didn't feel like an old, fat guy tonight."

Kathe M. Campbell

Diner's Club

Eating out has become a way of life in our fast-paced society, no longer just the occasional treat. Whether it's to avoid kitchen duty or to celebrate a special event, many meals are eaten at restaurants. For the weight-conscious, ordering from the menu can be a potential minefield. But, fear not, you can still eat out and enjoy your meal. Try incorporating just a few of these tips into your next dining experience, and eating out can please your palate without wrecking your waistline.

Begin with a starter. Then order another. There's your meal. The appetizer's smaller portions allow you variety in your diet as well as potentially fewer calories than if you opted for a traditional entrée with side dishes.

Ask for what you want. Don't be afraid to make special requests (politely, of course) so your meal is exactly what you want it to be.

Remember "G.B.S." Choose grilled, baked, broiled and steamed foods as often as you can. Try to steer clear of fried foods or creamy or cheesy sauces.

Don't go hungry. Have a healthy snack beforehand so you're not ravenous by the time you're seated. Two good options to defeat hunger pangs are apples or clear soup.

The doggy bag is your friend. Practice makes perfect, especially with portion control. I've actually used this method myself and stretched one meal into three. Don't trust your willpower to let you only eat a small portion? Ask your waiter to box up half of your meal. They might even keep it in the kitchen for you until you're ready to go. Be on the lookout; some chains will offer half-sizes of their meals.

Get your priorities straight. What would make the meal most memorable for you? Is there a house specialty you're dying to have? Or maybe their signature dessert? Pick one thing to build your meal around. Then go lightly with everything else. That means not having appetizers, soups, main course, bread and dessert. Now is the time to play favorites.

Try take-out. Practically and dietwise I've found you run into fewer temptations with take-out. You can add your lower-fat condiments like butter, sour cream and salad dressing to whatever you order and you won't be seduced by something not on your plan.

Beware of empty calories. Don't have wine just because everyone else is having a cocktail or it's happy hour. Would you rather have that drink or save calories for a special dessert? Likewise, if you're not wild about the bread, pass it on.

Order a special. If you're going to treat your-self, try something out of the ordinary that you can't get everywhere. Save the cheeseburger and fries for another time.

Lay off the sauce. Beware of anything cooked in butter, cheese or cream. If you simply can't have it without it, try getting it on the side.

Go fish. Most of the time, seafood, depending on the preparation, is less caloric and lower in cholesterol and fat than meat and pasta. It's especially good prepared following the "G.B.S." system.

Try a fill-up. On veggies, that is. Include veg-etables as integral parts of your meals when-ever possible. They help fill you up and meet your nutritional requirements. This is a great opportunity to try an exotic vegetable or one that you would never prepare at home due to time constraints, picky eaters or some other excuse. Otherwise, choose a salad, going easy on dressing and high-calorie toppings, or a vegetable-based soup.

Remember the "F" word. (Not that one!) During your meal, focus on friends and family, not feasting. It's not your last meal, so enjoy your company and the conversation.

Tricia Finch

Sit-Ups Till Your Eyes Pop Out

Worry is a misuse of the imagination.

Dan Zadra

The day was glorious, warm and fresh, the sky a clear Wedgwood blue. I was out for my morning run through the forest preserve, feeling vibrant and strong, breathing in the smell of new leaves and sunlit air. My electric-orange running shorts were cut high, showing a lot of leg, the black jog-bra cut low, showing a lot of skin.

When my shoelace came untied, I crouched to retie it. That's when I saw it. A fold of dimply flesh hanging over the waistband of my shorts. I gasped and shot up, arms high as if being robbed, looking at my belly. It was gone. *Oh, thank heavens,* I thought, it had just been a hideous hallucination. So I bent to finish tying the shoe, and there was the blasted thing again.

I had been blessed with thin genes and was one of those women who other women regarded with envy as I packed away unladylike mounds of food and never gained an ounce. I naively thought it would last forever and I would die an old woman with firm breasts, a tight butt and flat stomach.

The offending flesh shocked and appalled me, and I knew I'd have to get really serious now, so along with running, I took up aerobics, step-classes, spinning and Pilates. I started strength training and a new routine of leg lifts, curls and squats. I bought an Ab-Blaster.

At brunch one day I laid out my new exercise regimen to my friend Judi.

"This has to be obsessive-compulsive disorder," Judi pronounced. "You already look too good. Here, eat some of my eggs Benedict, you sicko." She pushed the gooey plate toward me. "If you get any better, I can't be friends with you any more."

Judi's idea of exercise was getting out of bed in the morning, and her idea of a healthy diet was a green salad and Diet Coke with her fettuccine Alfredo and chocolate mousse.

"I have to work on my stomach," I said. "I want six-pack abs."

"Hah!" Judi said. "I can just see it: you, in an ad in the back of a women's magazine, seventy years old, face wrinkled like linen on a hot day, but you're standing there in a string bikini, all buffed out with those six-pack abs."

"That won't happen," I said. "I'll have had a facelift before the photo shoot." I dipped a piece of pineapple in low-fat yogurt but felt faint from the aroma of eggs Benedict wafting up my nostrils.

"You're fifty years old. You can't get a six-pack when you're over fifty unless you go to a liquor store."

"Sure I can," I said. "I just have to work harder."

"Didn't we always say we were going to grow old gracefully?"

"Yeah, when we were fifteen. We also said we'd never spank our kids in the grocery store and we'd never use a cell phone and we'd never turn into our mothers."

Judi shrugged, pulled back her plate and took a large bite, dripping with hollandaise.

"Look at Cher," I continued. "Look at Goldie Hawn. Every time I see Goldie's flat stomach in one of her little body-skimming evening gowns at the Academy Awards, I want to scream. She's older than I am. If she has a flat stomach, I can, too."

"Those women spend more on plastic surgery than we spend on our mortgages. Get real. No one's exempt. We're all getting old. Let's do it with some dignity."

I considered Judi's words as I immersed myself in my new training program. What does aging gracefully mean, I wondered one day as I did twenty extra squats. Letting yourself go? Giving up? I ran an extra mile that day.

On the day I finished fifty crunches and thirty-five leg lifts, I heard Judi's voice in my head: "No one's exempt. We're all getting old. Let's do it with dignity." And when I finally worked up to sixty-two reps on the Ab-Blaster (shooting for one hundred) I collapsed, gasping, wondering where this was getting me. The belly-roll was still there in spite of my punishing efforts. I could probably do sit-ups until my eyes popped out and that flab would sit there, unperturbed, mocking me.

I lay on the floor, mopping my sweat-soaked hair. And then I got up, grabbed the Ab-Blaster furiously as if it had bitten me and took it out to the trash. I vowed to accept being fifty-something with all its consequences: excess hair where I didn't want it, thinning hair where I did, drooping breasts, sagging butt and the inability to focus on my eyelashes as I tried to coat them with mascara. I would be happy with who I was and how I looked now. I would. I really would.

I opened a Diet Coke and drank thirstily, looking out the kitchen window, breathing in the smell of the sunlit air. Something moved by the garbage can and I frowned and squinted. Someone was picking up the Ab-Blaster. Hesitating for only a split second I rushed to the door and threw it open with a thwack!

"Hey!" I shouted, running out. "Leave that alone. I need that!"

Samantha Hoffman

Chocolate Is Not the Enemy

He can inspire a group only if he himself is filled with confidence and hope of success.

Floyd V. Filson

It wasn't yet 7:00 in the morning and already I was chain-eating lime chili tortilla chips. I stood at the kitchen counter, emotionally hung-over from yet another fight with my boyfriend. I was crunching the anger, salting the wounds. Crunching and salting with bites of chocolate for good measure. I couldn't stop. Even the tortilla chip bag had a wickedly furious crinkle. I couldn't eat fast enough to block the tension of not wanting to abandon my relationship, not knowing how to go on. I was broken, a whir of helplessness, powerlessness. This echoed my drinking days. Twelve years I'd been sober. How did I get this way with food? This had to stop. Had to stop! What had been an occasional binge followed by days of deprivation had become a near-daily nightmare.

A prayer flashed through my mind, one that my friend Marti Matthews shares in her book, *Pain: The Challenge and the Gift.* It goes like this: "Help! Help! Help! Help! Help!"

Which, she suggests, can be repeated with hands thrown in the air.

I repeated it silently all the way to a breakfast with one of my best friends, a bearer of wonders and wise words. While I collected myself, she whipped out a flyer from her bag and slapped it on my empty plate. "Taking Your Own Shape: Explore Your Relationship with Food and Body," it said.

What? Oh my God. The most important part of praying for help is recognizing it when it arrives. Darn, I'd have to go.

The class was intimate and scary. Six women sitting on couches. That first night, I felt like someone who'd arrived from another planet with a "Waiting for Instructions" note pinned to my soul. Please tell me what to do and when to do it. Give me the whole calories in/calories out regime with a few collages thrown in to express my creativity and no one will get hurt. Now!

Instead, we talked. And we listened. We talked about our bodies—what it felt like to live in them. We shared our love and lack of love for others and ourselves. We set no weight-loss goals. We suffered no weekly weigh-ins or calculations of the foods we ate, and in what proportions. Got no stickers for eating right. Or scowls for eating wrong.

In fact, Dr. Becky Coleman, our teacher, said there was no right or wrong, only alive and less alive. She needn't have told us. She radiated acceptance. She embodied an invitation to a whole new level of living that was spacious and expressive. She'd weighed 300 pounds, not once, but twice. Eight years ago, she lost 170 pounds and has never found them again.

How strange. My body was a Frankenstein to me, out of control, hunted and feared by the villagers. Becky practiced compassionate experimentation. Explore your weight. Don't condemn it. Perhaps hunger was a message from your deep, wise self. What if your body generously expressed what you were afraid to? Well, if my body was speaking, it was mumbling, that's for sure. Maybe because its mouth was full.

One evening we introduced our "Favorite Food Friends" to each other. A vegetarian brought a huge plate of steak and french fries. I showed my old faithful Ben and Jerry's Chubby Hubby ice cream. Chocolate-covered peanut butter–filled pretzels tucked into vanilla ice cream. I'd met Chubby Hubby years ago when my then live-in boyfriend moved away. It was everything: salty, crunchy, soft, sweet. Thanks to Ben and Jerry's planet-friendly ethics, I could save myself and the world at the same time.

"You say you crave variety," said Becky. "Interesting variety in that carton." She invited us to experiment with our food friends. Did we reach for them in anger? Sorrow? What would happen if we held the tension that triggered the craving just for a moment?

The next time Chubby Hubby called, I paused with spoon in hand. I let my body experience the ache for peace with my lover. Then I ate the ice cream.

Instead of slapping my thighs and cursing my will-power, I became curious. So there really were emotions trying to emerge between bites. My body relished the pauses from chips and chocolate. Attention at last! I began to enjoy feeling fluid and elegant instead of leaden. Twenty pounds fell away. Discovering that my cravings, my clenched heart, my anxious belly had answers for me was like being lost and panicky in the woods and discovering the trees could speak. Now when trees speak, I listen.

Jan Henrikson

A Can of Peas and
a Jog Around the Block

*Nothing in the world can take the place of
persistence.*

Calvin Coolidge

One summer day, a dozen years ago, I stood at my living room window and watched two women walk by on the sidewalk. They were both young mothers and each pushed a stroller while holding a toddler about the same size as Dana, my then two-year-old daughter. It struck me how alike the women looked—heavy and slow, with untucked, oversized T-shirts covering ample butts and bellies. Then my window became a mirror, and I saw myself. I looked just like them.

In that instant, as I stood there in my untucked, oversized T-shirt and elastic-waist shorts, I knew I had to make some changes. God was hitting me over the head with a giant foam hammer: "This is an epiphany, Lori. Run with it." And that, more or less, is what I did.

I'd always been a tiny person, never needing to exercise and able to eat whatever, whenever, and remain trim and

petite. I'd even come out the other end of my first pregnancy smaller than when I went into it. I'd had a hard time
just holding onto my first child, a boy. After seven months
of nausea, projectile rejection of almost all food save
Cheerios and Dannon yogurt, and a stint in the hospital
hooked to a nasogastric tube that delivered protein drink
through my nostrils to my stomach, my Adam greeted the
world two months early—four pounds and able to fit in
the palm of my husband's hand. When we took our tiny
fighter home after his stay in intensive care, I weighed five
pounds less than I'd weighed in high school.

Dana stayed in the womb a week beyond the due date.
While I carried Dana, she and I ate. About every twenty
minutes. With Adam, I felt sick if I ate. With Dana, I felt sick
if I didn't. I embarked on a nine-month, nonstop eating
orgy. Steak, peanut butter, baked potatoes with sour
cream, hot fudge sundaes. Deli meat, frozen pizza, Cheez-
Its by the boxful. Oreos, burritos, chocolate and butterscotch pudding smothered in Reddi-wip. I slept with a
loaf of bread next to the bed.

When Dana was born, healthy and beautiful, I was big.
And stayed big. And pretended I wasn't. Had God sent
the two strolling mothers any earlier, I wouldn't have
been ready to receive the message. Being in denial awhile
had allowed me to keep eating doughnuts, corned-beef
hash and bacon while rationalizing the weight gain as a
normal, perfectly acceptable stage of motherhood.

Upon my epiphany, I resolved to effect a wholesale,
cold-turkey conversion. I knew exactly what I had to do:
eat less, eat well, move more. Forever. And it's the forever
part that made the whole thing easier to swallow.

Were I to put myself "on a diet," I knew I would fail, ultimately if not right away. I needed to replace "diet," a short-
term, emergency-infused concept, with "life," hopefully
long and good. I would never be on a diet. I'd be on life.

This gave me more time to succeed. A diet would demand results in a few weeks. Life gave me more time. All the time in the world.

A diet would have me devote a finite number of weeks or months to counting, measuring and portioning, allowing me an extra gram of sugar here and there so I could live a little. Life, on the other hand said, "Don't live a little, live fully. Use common sense to live well. You know what's good and what's not, so, most of the time, just do what's good."

And a diet would address only what I took in. But life offered the chance to play with energy, experiment with taking it in and burning it off. A diet held no challenge: Here, eat this measured thing. Life said, "Have some fun. See what happens when you eat a little and burn a little. Or eat a lot and burn a little. Or eat a little and burn a lot. Or eat a lot and burn a lot." What fun! Like being a scientist. Diet? Every day is grapefruit. Life? Every day is different.

So I banished "diet" from my mind-set and lexicon and focused on life. I resolved to do three things: center my meals around plants, choose healthy calories over bad or empty ones, and move for at least twenty minutes a day.

When the time came for my first postconversion meal, I opened the fridge. I wanted to plant-center my plate, but there wasn't a fresh fruit or vegetable in that whole Kenmore. I opened the cupboard and took down a can of peas. I found an onion, sautéed it in olive oil, threw in some chopped garlic and lemon juice and folded the mix into the peas. I poured a tall glass of orange juice, sat down on my deck and tucked into this humble, healthy lunch that would change my life.

The next morning, I dug out an old pair of sneakers, pulled on my elastic-waist shorts and oversized T-shirt and went outside to move. I started out walking but soon found myself lifting my feet high enough off the ground to approximate a rude form of entry-level shuffle-jogging. That first day, I made it once around the block. I felt like I was going to die, but I knew I'd run the race of my life.

Now, after years of salads, fruit, fish, chicken, whole grains and the occasional Oreo or Dairy Queen cone, I wear high school–size jeans and have long since given away my elastic-waist shorts.

And that energy experiment? My favorite take in/burn off combination is "eat a lot and burn a lot." That's what I do when I train for a marathon. I'm preparing for my sixth.

Lori Hein

Take Two

Patience and perseverance have a magical effect before which difficulties disappear and obstacles vanish.

John Quincy Adams

There is something about everyone they're not happy with. Maybe it's their weight, hair, eyes or skin color, their shoe size, job situation or relationships—any number of things.

For me, it's always been my weight. When I hit puberty I sprouted a chest, a butt and a little gut all at once. I became aware of things I never had before, in places I never thought of before. I became increasingly self-conscious.

Some girls chose not to eat. I chose the opposite and began eating too much. My appetite sky-rocketed, but I looked fine, until I hit eighteen. Then it was as if gravity had something against me at an early age. I was making bad eating decisions, was depressed and cared way too much about what people thought of me.

Eventually my weight became an obstacle in the way of happiness—or so I thought.

It took many years of these bad eating habits for me to end up considerably overweight. I would diet, crash diet, nose-dive diet; if there was a diet out there, I was on it. I tried about everything but eating tofu with tweezers! (Don't think I didn't consider it though.) And I would lose weight, only to gain it right back, and then some.

A constant frustration for me was the emphasis that society placed on being thin. Thin is beautiful. To those of us who aren't, we must resolve to lose weight and be healthy and live happily ever after. That moment of fortitude vanishes the minute the delivery boy, holding the extra-large pepperoni pizza with extra cheese, rings the doorbell and you think, *Well, I paid for it; I might as well eat it!* which is exactly what I would do. Then I would feel terrible about my lack of self-control and cry.

Of course I comforted myself with a double-dark chocolate candy bar, or two or three, which worked until I read the nutrition label. Imagine my shock to discover my delusion about chocolate being a vegetable. Hey, it comes from a bean, and beans are vegetables, aren't they? The justification and rationalizations never end.

On a day I resolved to lose weight and be healthy, I would consume over 4,000 calories! I know I was in the junk food line a little too long when they handed out those metabolisms, but even the women who pack it away and stay tiny wouldn't last long at that rate. I was living in an endless cycle of guilt, unhappiness and failure.

I would make jokes about myself so I'd feel less self-conscious about the way I looked. I would tell people, "I should put stickers on my holster hips that say, 'Caution, wide turns.'" Or how about this one: "I get applause when I run in gym class. My thighs slap together so loud it sounds like everyone's clapping." After all, my attitude is based on 10 percent of what life hands me, and 90 percent of how I react to what life hands me.

It didn't occur to me until later that, like almost everything in life, happiness is a choice. I made some bad choices in the food I ate, and how much of it. Now I have to reverse the process. In the end, it isn't about crash diets or what society thinks—it's about learning to have a diet. Everything we eat is a diet, and one secret is to keep things in proportion. Another is choosing to be happy with what you have—no matter how much more of it you've been given.

God, my husband, and the prayers of many family and friends are the reason I'm able to put life into a different perspective today. Society doesn't define happiness—especially mine. I no longer let it. What we do with our lives and bodies is up to us. I had to change my attitude before I could change my eating habits. There are certain things about myself that I can't change, but the things I can, I am learning to be less obsessive about and more patient with.

I'm still in a weight-loss process and will be for a long time, but now when I answer that door and find an extra-large pepperoni pizza with extra cheese waiting, I'll have two slices instead of four—and choose to be happy that I had any at all.

Karen A. Bakhazi

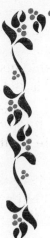

Poached Eggs au Gratin

MAKES 2 SERVINGS
EACH SERVING: 19 GRAMS PROTEIN, TRACE CARBOHYDRATE

1 tablespoon white vinegar
4 eggs
2 tablespoons grated Parmesan cheese
2 teaspoons chopped fresh parsley

In a deep medium skillet, bring 2 inches of water and vinegar to a boil over high heat.

Reduce heat to simmer. Crack an egg into a small bowl and tip gently into boiling water. Repeat with all eggs.

Cover skillet and cook 3 minutes for soft yolks, 5 minutes for firmer yolks. Using a slotted spoon, remove eggs from water and drain thoroughly.

Sprinkle with grated Parmesan cheese and fresh parsley. Serve immediately.

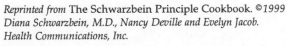

Reprinted from The Schwarzbein Principle Cookbook. ©1999
Diana Schwarzbein, M.D., Nancy Deville and Evelyn Jacob.
Health Communications, Inc.

You Choose, You Lose

Destiny is not a matter of chance; it is a matter of choice. It is not a thing to be waited for; it is a thing to be achieved.

William Jennings Bryan

"I've had it. I'm sick and tired of saying I can't have something," I complained to my best friend Linda. "I can't have chocolate cake. I can't have ice cream. I can't have a yummy éclair. Is there anything I can have?"

"You can have lots of things," she said.

"Yeah, right. You're not the one trying to lose weight. The whole world is filled with things that are off-limits." I sulked in my chair as I read the lunch menu in the restaurant.

Pastrami on rye. Cheeseburger. Tuna melt.

Roast beef au jus. French fries. Onion rings.

Cheesy broccoli soup. New England clam chowder.

Double-fudge brownies. Blueberry cheesecake.

The choices were endless.

As a teenager I could eat anything I wanted and as much as I wanted. Not anymore. Now I step on the scale every morning and peek at the numbers, hoping they haven't gone higher than the day before. I'm happy if I haven't gained and elated if I've lost even half a pound. It's a daily struggle and I'm tired of fighting. I'm even more tired of that word "can't."

There are so many things in life I just can't control. How tall I am (I always wanted to be short like my sister). My boss (I wish he'd save the big projects for Monday instead of Friday afternoons). The high cost of living (I wonder if I'll ever be able to retire). I have no power over so many areas of my life. Is there something I could take control of?

Then the light bulb went off in my head, one of those "ah ha" moments when it all comes together. There was something I could control—my own mind and my own decisions.

I did have a choice in this one area, the area of what I chose to eat. I could pick something I knew would be good for me, or I could pick something that wasn't in line with my goals. It was all a matter of choice. And it was all up to me.

Linda's voice brought me out of my thoughts. "How about the BLT? Or is that something you can't have?"

"You know what? Starting right now, right this minute, I'm not going to say 'can't' anymore." I sat up straight in my chair. "I'm going to say what I choose to have instead."

"Sounds like a good plan to me," Linda said. "So what are you having?"

"I'm choosing the Chinese chicken salad and I'm asking for the dressing on the side."

"Sounds terrific. But you can't have a soda with that, right?" she said. "Oops, I said can't. I'm sorry."

"That's okay; it will take a while to get used to it. But to answer you, I'm choosing ice water with a slice of lemon today."

I felt great when I came out of the restaurant after lunch. Not only did I not feel bloated from eating too much, but the salad filled me up just fine. And most of all, I felt more in control of my mind and of my eating habits.

It was something I could choose, and I love the feeling of power I have in that.

B. J. Taylor

Whatever I Want

You cannot make yourself feel something you do not feel, but you can make yourself do right in spite of your feelings.

Pearl S. Buck

Two months into my new life as a gastric bypass patient, I have begun a journey into my past to see if I can answer some of the questions I have about what led me to the 385-pound, high-water mark in my life. As this new tool has allowed me to begin shedding the weight, gain confidence and overcome my failure mentality, I have realized that what it hasn't done is to banish my mental cravings for food. This is not totally unexpected. I knew from the start that weight-loss surgery was no magic pill or sorcerer's spell that would make all of my fat issues disappear in a puff of smoke. But the hope is always there, isn't it?

So, as I sit here, watching the weight disappear, notching new holes in my old belt and trying to ignore the siren song of the kitchen, I'm also looking back over the years to try to find out what hole in my psyche I have tried for so long to fill with food. For years I've blamed my hunger on a slow metabolism, super-size stomach and a faulty telephone line between my belly and my brain. Now that my stomach holds no more than a couple of ounces, and I know that I've recently filled that with dense protein, any feelings of hunger cannot be related to my belly. In fact, the sense of fullness that I'm feeling even as I type would suggest that, were I to give in to the impulse to grab a snack, I would probably find myself hugging the toilet in the near future, as all engines reversed.

So, into the past . . . as a child I grew up in a poverty-stricken neighborhood. I can easily recall weeks when our only food was potatoes and government-granted bricks of processed cheese. Breakfast, lunch and dinner . . . potatoes and cheese. In all fairness, I have since spent time in countries where this abundance would be reason for celebration and now understand what a blessing from God it was to have food, any food, on the table when so many in this world do not. However, that reasoning has little impact on the mind of a child or the mental pathways and habits that are formed during this most influential time of our lives.

Over the years life improved, but only slightly. It wasn't until I was out of high school that I lived a life completely free of government financial aid. We were "poor," and that was a message that echoed both from our bank statements and from the innermost parts of our self-image. By the time I was ten or twelve, I had ceased to ask for anything beyond the most basic needs. The mantra in our apartment was "We don't have the money for . . ." Regardless of the object of desire, the answer was always the same.

Lest there be any jumping to conclusions, I want to make it clear that this WAS the reality. I had no miserly mother who saved every extra penny for her own clothing, booze or cigarettes. Mom did the best she could with very, very little. When she said we could not afford it, it was because there were not enough pennies in the cookie jar to buy bread, much less the new style of jeans, the latest record or the new Nikes that all the "cool" kids were wearing. Thus, I became used to the mantra and tried to keep my chin up despite the taunts of other kids and the deep-seated sense of being less than my peers. The only thing that saved me from serious psychological damage, at least in my opinion, was that I grew up in a home rich with love. Positive reinforcement, loving touch and acceptance were as plentiful as cash was not.

So, starting at an age younger than I can remember now, I began my own mantra. A handful of words that represented a respite from the unfairness of our privation. For every gift-laden store window, every school trip that left without me, every trip to the secondhand store, I repeated these words: "When I grow up, I will have whatever I want." This was the magic spell. The hope of things unseen that helped me survive on potatoes, cheese and two-dollar tennis shoes from Kmart. "Whatever I want."

Twenty years have passed since I became able to work and earn my own money and provide things for both myself and my loved ones that we hadn't had for so long. What greater joy than to walk into the burger restaurant and order one . . . no, TWO . . . of the biggest burgers they had, as well as the largest french fries and the super-sized drink. To look at the menu and present myself with "whatever I want." No one could tell me we didn't have the money; why, I could pull the bills right from my own wallet and order everything on the menu (and sometimes it seems that I tried).

What greater proof that the days of want and lack were gone forever—to banish that fear and self-loathing—than to swagger down the junk food aisle and grab all the jumbo bags of chips, all the Oreo cookies (and not the cheap, stale knock-offs) that I wanted and toss them into the cart? Big, colorful bottles of Coke were far more satisfying than ten-for-a-dollar packages of generic Kool-aid. Delivery pizza was expensive. Poor people couldn't afford to have an extra large with everything on it brought to their door, right? Therefore every call to Dominoes reinforced the proof that I could have whatever I wanted. And every extra burger, every ice cream cone, every jumbo bag of chips was a time machine that whispered comfort back over the years to a little boy sitting at a worn Formica table with nothing on his plate but a baked potato.

Every dollar spent, every mouthful of food was a silent cry that I would not spend the rest of my life as it had started out, in poverty and want. Deep in my mind, in my heart, did I think I was doing it for him? Did I really believe that every overindulgence on the part of the teenage me, and later the young-adult me, could somehow justify the faith that a little-boy me had placed in his helplessly frustrated mantra? You bet I did. You see, I owed it to him. The only way to justify his lack was in my own abundance. The greater my excess, the less he haunted my dreams. And it had to be reproven every day, every hour, every time the opportunity arose to either deny myself (We don't have the money for . . .) or to slake my hunger, thirst and desire (whatever I want).

I was thirty-five years old and growing rapidly toward 400 pounds before a stronger, more insistent voice finally drowned out the mantra. This voice was the fear of death. Within three months I had been diagnosed with diabetes, high blood pressure and a cholesterol level so high that it couldn't be charted. I could barely cross the room without losing my breath. At home I had a wonderful, loving wife who cared for and supported me, a church full of people who I loved and who loved me, and the first steps taken toward my dream of being a novelist. The only thing that stood in the way of being a healthy, happy, successful man was a little boy in a dingy apartment kitchen repeating over and over, "Whatever I want. . . ."

And by some miracle, by the earnest prayers of my loved ones, I finally listened to a new voice. Another year has passed since then and I'm now several weeks out from my Roux en-Y (RNY) surgery. Forty-five pounds have disappeared since the operation, as well as forty before, and another pound follows almost daily. But I still hear the continuous calling from the pantry and refrigerator, and the whispers as I drive past the seemingly innumerable fast-food joints between my work and home.

So I must remember whose voice it is that I'm hearing. Food has no voice, I remind myself; it is deaf, dumb and dead, a collection of elements and nutrients that cannot act on me unless I act on them first. No, food does not call to me. I call to me—a younger, lesser version of myself who only understands that he is being told, once again, what he cannot have. I struggle to teach him a new mantra, as I struggle to justify his deprivation: "When I grow up, I will have whatever I need." And after all these years I begin to realize that maybe that is what he really meant.

Perry P. Perkins

Finally, Success—A New Me!

The secret of health for both mind and body is not to mourn for the past, worry about the future, or anticipate troubles, but to live in the present moment wisely and earnestly.

Buddha

No one except my doctor really knew how much I weighed. Every time I had to renew my driver's license and was asked if anything had changed, I said "No" and wondered if I could go to jail for lying to the secretary of state. Now, for the first time since I was about thirty, I'm legal.

I used to claim my excess weight was postpregnancy weight, but since I'm now sixty-one with sons thirty-five and thirty-six and actually gained only twelve pounds with each pregnancy, it seems a bit ridiculous.

I've gone to Weight Watchers, TOPS and other weight-loss groups. I succumbed to every magazine at the checkout counters that promised to share the secret of losing weight. I used incentives, like "the class reunion is coming up, I need to lose forty pounds in two weeks."

Having been in the healthcare field, I knew how to eat properly and be healthy. I knew all the dangers of being overweight. But only when the scare of things that "could" go wrong actually became a reality did I wake up and smell the Columbian brew.

Each time I had a physical and passed (and I'm an over-achiever, so I'm used to passing tests), I said a prayer of thanks and promised God I would give him a hand and help out in the being healthy department. I guess he got tired of listening to that tune because one day he threw me a real curveball.

My blood sugar was a little elevated, so my doctor ordered a glucose tolerance test. I'll be darned if I didn't flunk a test! She said, "Well, you didn't stop at pre-diabetes —you're diabetic." The date was November 15, 2004.

I went home totally scared to death, angry and positive that any good quality of my life was indeed over. I read the booklets my doctor had given me, went to the pharmacy and purchased the little blood test meter. My husband took me out to dinner, where I ate like Miss Piggy on the way to the bacon factory.

I began counting carbs and testing the next day. Maybe because I hate math, I hate to count anything—calories, carbs, fat grams—losing ten pounds seemed like such a huge task. But I was determined. Not determined halfway, like before when I'd lose five pounds and gain them right back, but really determined.

Even before my consultation with the dietician at the diabetes clinic, I'd lost seven pounds. By the first of the year, I'd lost seventeen pounds—OVER THE HOLIDAYS! My blood sugar dropped immediately with the slightest weight loss.

When I realized counting carbs was easier than I thought, it became a way of life. I knew what I could eat. I ate three meals a day with three small snacks in between if I wanted, which usually I didn't. I expected the dietician to give me a whole list of foods I could never eat again. He didn't. It was all about portion control. What a concept! Of course, I already knew that half a box of spaghetti wasn't really a serving. But, come on, two ounces of pasta! Show me someone content with that and I'll show you a fuzzy little rodent in a cage with an exercise wheel. But, guess what? I am content with that.

I enjoy my food now more than ever because I'm busy tasting and enjoying it and not just shoveling it in. When asked my secret, I say, "I'm eating for one, not for Sandi and a third world country."

I was still fat on my sixtieth birthday. The number stuck in my throat. I couldn't even say it. Now, as I approach sixty-two this summer, I can say it with ease because I don't look or feel my age. As I listen to talk of diets and weight struggles, I'm amazed at how truly easy it ultimately was.

So, that's the end of my story, my fat story that is. This is the beginning of the NEW me story and my new healthy life. I wear a size 6 jeans—real zip-up jeans now, not elastic-waist-fat-girl jeans. I work out at the health club three times a week (I started out at five to six times a week). I walk two miles and work out on the weight machines. I go to yoga classes. I eat what I want to— portion control. I've lost sixty pounds and feel twenty years younger. I have unlimited energy, and most important, my blood sugar is totally normal even when I go a little higher on the carbs once in a while.

I am healthy, energetic and happy. My doctor has changed my diagnosis, and she smiled when I said, "At my age, I want to be healthy and feel good. Looking good is the bonus."

Sandra L. Tatara

The Mirror Doesn't Lie

Keep the faculty of effort alive in you by a little gratuitous exercise every day.

William James

I was in the mall the other day, rushing to get errands done and pausing just for a second to shift packages from one arm to the other. For a fleeting moment, I got that feeling women are apt to get—a sense of being stared at, that a set of discerning eyes was looking and passing judgment. I shrugged the feeling off and continued on my way. When you're fifty-something and have looked fairly dowdy most of your adult life—not just in an encroaching golden age—you get used to the looks, or lack of them. When you're carrying more than a few extra pounds, you can find yourself teetering on a tightrope between people staring or drowning in a sea of invisibility.

Strangers pass judgment when you're obese. It may be as overt as a pointed finger or thoughtless laugh, or as subtle as pretending you don't exist. I remembered back. . . .

"Is there something I can help you with, ma'am?" There certainly was. The clerk was my age, a handsome man with wavy black hair and solid, angular features. I'd been patiently trying to get his attention for some help with a wallet I was selecting for a Christmas present.

It was near dinnertime, and the shop was pleasantly near-empty. The only shoppers were me: short, solid and rather hefty; and a girl my age then—perhaps twenty— with perfect flowing hair, perfect hands, chiseled legs and a body with the flesh secured firmly to the bone. She was lovely, and the clerk was smitten.

For what seemed like forever, I thumbed through wallets—now and then lifting my head with a smile, trying to make eye contact, to get his attention. It wasn't happening. Only when the "normal" girl was gone did he realize I needed his help.

And then he called me "ma'am." It was the first time that ever happened to me. When I left the shop and got to the safe place inside my car, where the windows steamed in the winter night, hot, embarrassed tears stung my cheeks.

And yet I did nothing about it. Except to maybe eat some more and gain an increasing amount of weight.

Decades passed, and layers and layers of fat enfolded me. I was far beyond even "ma'am" now. I was nearly asexual. I made fewer and fewer trips to shops—to public places in general. I was no longer hefty. I was huge. Walking around the block caught me out of breath and sent my knees into agonizing aches and spasms.

I knew if it kept on, I was going to die. A real, tangible, physical death. For a while, even with that reality in place, I shrugged off my destiny. It had been years since I looked into a mirror. People had stopped looking at me years ago, and I'd given it up for myself as well.

It was a dark, dark place.

I know exactly when the light came on. It was about a year ago, when sleeping at night was now no longer an option. Every time I lay down, it was difficult to breathe. Day and night, I walked the floors, exhausted, and now, finally, thoroughly afraid.

And then, it happened. In one on-a-whim, entirely out-of-character moment, I ventured out into a public place for the first time in a very long time—to the animal shelter. That's where Max found me. He was so very small for a shepherd/golden mix, and so very sick. I saw his face and forgot about my knees.

Max had no time for excuses. He needed medication every few hours, and because of the medicine, he needed more walks than a "normal" puppy. Because he also came with allergies, he needed to eat natural and healthy food And so, on another fine day, I found myself in the produce department instead of the ice cream aisle.

He grew strong and began to thrive, and so did I. More than a year passed, and I was down ten sizes. Max was home, I was sure, comfortably snoozing on the couch where he wasn't supposed to be, and I was at the mall, running errands and thinking about my past.

The shopping bags needed to be shifted, and again I stopped. Once more I felt the sensation that a pair of eyes was watching. This time, I held my head up and looked back.

What I saw jolted me. It was a woman, just about my age, short but easy on the eye, tanned and fit. I smiled, and she was smiling back.

I had stopped in front of a full-length mirror.

These days, the anguish is gone, along with the self-loathing and embarrassment, and I no longer fear my own reflection. Max has no problem looking into my eyes. Why, then, should I?

Candy Killion

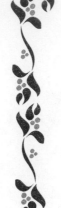

Ricotta-Stuffed Bell Peppers

MAKES 4 SERVINGS
EACH SERVING: 24 GRAMS PROTEIN, 11 GRAMS CARBOHYDRATE

4 bell peppers, cut in half lengthwise
1½ pounds whole ricotta cheese
2 eggs
½ cup chopped Kalamata olives
1 cup chopped raw walnuts
½ cup minced fresh parsley
2 tablespoons slivered fresh basil or
    2 teaspoons dried basil
1 tablespoon grated lemon zest
freshly ground black pepper to taste
⅔ cup Parmesan cheese

Preheat oven to 350°. Cut bell peppers in half and remove seeds. In a large skillet, bring 2 cups water to a boil. Add bell peppers, reduce heat to low and simmer until just tender, about 8 to 10 minutes. Remove from pan, drain and set aside.

In a medium bowl, combine ricotta cheese, eggs, olives, walnuts, parsley, basil, lemon zest and black pepper. Mix well with a fork. Mound into pepper halves. Sprinkle with Parmesan cheese. Place in an ovenproof baking dish and add water to ¼-inch depth in pan to prevent burning. Bake until heated through, about 20 to 30 minutes. Place under broiler briefly to brown top.

Reprinted from The Schwarzbein Principle Cookbook. ©1999
Diana Schwarzbein, M.D., Nancy Deville and Evelyn Jacob.
Health Communications, Inc.

The Thighs Have It

I was leafing through a magazine where there was a before-and-after picture of a woman who went from a size 5 to a size 3 by liposuction. Was she serious? I've cooked bigger turkeys than her "before" picture.

Erma Bombeck

After a workout at the health club, my friend and I are in the dressing room, getting ready for work. She gathers together hairbrush and makeup, goes to one of the many large mirrors and instantly frowns. "I hate the way I look," she mutters. The woman next to her is also frowning, tugging fretfully on what looks to me like enviable, long golden hair. An olive-skinned, raven-haired beauty wearing a black silk pantsuit scowls when she turns sideways to analyze the pooch of her stomach. I'd like to cover all the mirrors, so all these beautiful women who are muttering dark and gloomy mantras of "too fat, too saggy, too flabby, too wrinkly" could have a break.

Just recently I had a lesson in mirror watching and learned that, like Alice, what I see in the looking glass is often just a reflection of mood and interpretation. Here's what happened. My husband, Ron, and I were at a California resort, complete with a wonderful swimming pool, lovely, natural hot mineral springs, palm trees, brilliant bougainvillea flowers and lots of chairs for lounging, reading and dreaming. I had never been in such a gorgeous and peaceful spot, and I was thoroughly enjoying myself. I emerged from a glorious swim in the heated pool and went to the bathroom. In the dressing area, a full-length mirror surprised me. Without thinking, I glanced at myself, dripping in my bathing suit. My thighs jiggled and sagged. What? How was that possible? Wasn't I exercising a lot and eating properly? I could have chocolate as part of a healthy diet, right? I felt a stab of despair; my thighs were abandoning me. I walked out and Ron said, "What's wrong?"

"My thighs are jiggly," I said.

Ron looked carefully at the offending appendages. "That's true," he said. (I have tried to teach him that honesty is not always the best policy, but obviously that concept had not sunk in.) "But I still love you."

"Thank you," I said. I slunk over to a lounge chair, wishing he had said, "Gee honey, your thighs look great to me!" I put a towel over my legs and opened my book to page 103. But the sun was too bright, a bee was too close to me and I couldn't concentrate. My mind was knotted up in images of ugliness and aging. I decided to get back into the hot pool and let the warmth and wet soothe me. A woman with a lovely silver ponytail and a glowing tan was luxuriating in the water. "You must eat right and work out," she said as I approached. "You have a wonderful figure."

I stopped and stared at her. "Really?" I said.

"Oh yes, you look great."

"Really?" I said. "Are you sure?"

"Of course," she said calmly. "I'm very sure."

I eased myself into the water and touched my thighs. I

noticed how easy it was to hear Ron's affirmation of my flabby thighs and how hard it was to take in this woman's compliment. *I look great*, I said to myself, tasting the words like they were something delicious. In less than an hour, I had seen the subjectivity of physical looks. After all, it's a lonely business, worrying about your upper legs. It's a culturally induced trauma, and I didn't have to embrace it.

As I sank into the steaming water, I had a radical thought: What if I decided I looked great every day? My spirits would rise, my face would glow, and I would feel strong and happy. Which means I would probably look great. And that is what I am trying to do.

Deborah H. Shouse

Mirror, Mirror on the Wall

Forty-three percent of men and 56 percent of women are unhappy about their overall appearance. They are concerned about flaws in their skin, hair, face and weight.

However, some people worry so much about their appearance that it leads to serious problems in their relationships with others and makes it impossible to carry on a normal daily routine.

People suffering with body dysmorphic disorder (BDD), also referred to as body image disorder, are so preoccupied with a distorted idea of what they look like that thoughts about their perceived flaws consume them.

Often the "flaw" doesn't even exist or is blown entirely out of proportion, but someone suffering with BDD does not see the same person in the mirror that everyone else sees.

The American Psychiatric Association estimates that BDD affects one in fifty people, more often girls in their teens or early twenties.

If you need help with BDD, contact a qualified mental health professional. For more information on BDD, read Katharine Phillips's groundbreaking book, *Broken Mirror: Understanding and Treating Body Dysmorphic Disorder.*

Where Money Meets Resolutions

Money can't buy you happiness, but it does bring you a more pleasant form of misery.

Spike Milligan

The one thing I hate more than exercising is spending money. That explains why my fingers trembled as I signed a one-year contract and then a credit card slip for membership to a women's fitness center. Although I had resolved to get fit, my "frugal" genes were not happy.

After a brief tussle, the manager pried the slip away from my unwilling fingers. "You're going to love it here," she chirped. "Worth every penny."

"It better be," I muttered. As I debated snatching the slip back and making a run for it, one look at the chiseled muscles on her size 4 body told me I'd be lucky to get halfway out of the chair before she tackled me.

I consoled myself with the thought that if I gave up my daily coffee, I could afford to work out. On the other hand, caffeine had been a close, personal friend for years. Did I really want to turn my back on it now?

I was debating the pros and cons when the manager's voice interrupted my thoughts.

"We have a fantastic introductory personal trainer package. At just $400 for ten sessions, we're practically giving it away." She leaned in and lowered her voice. "I shouldn't tell you, but the price is going up next week."

"Four hundred dollars?" my voice came out as a loud croak.

"I know. Unbelievable. Should I sign you up?" Not waiting for my answer, she took out another credit card slip and wrote in the date.

My mouth opened but no words came out. I tried to figure out what else I would have to give up to cover the additional costs. Probably food. On the other hand, that would make losing weight a lot faster.

I was still adding figures in my head when she thrust a pen into my hand. My fingers automatically wrapped around it. Dazed by the kaleidoscope of numbers whirling in my brain, I signed my name for the third time in five minutes.

With Houdini-like sleight of hand, she whisked the slip from under my hand but couldn't pry the pen from my death grip. "Why don't you keep the pen," she said. "Our gift to you."

A few minutes later, still clutching the pen, I was back on the street. Did I really want to do this? Did the contract have an escape clause? Resolutions are one thing. But actually committing myself to a year's membership and ten personal training sessions, not to mention their locker and towel service, was another.

I'd spent over $800 and hadn't lost a pound or gained an ounce of muscle yet. The only thing lighter was my bank account.

The next two months were hard. When tempted to slack off from my workout routine, I gazed at my bank balance and pushed myself out the front door. By March, as I felt healthier and stronger, I surprised myself by looking forward to my workouts.

That was last January. Since then, I've purchased two more training packages and renewed my membership. And my fingers barely trembled when I signed on the dotted line. I've lost weight, dropped two pants sizes and gained muscle. I might not be able to beat the manager at arm wrestling, but at least now I could give her a run for my money.

As for the pen, I keep it as a reminder that sometimes spending money is a good investment—in yourself.

Harriet Cooper

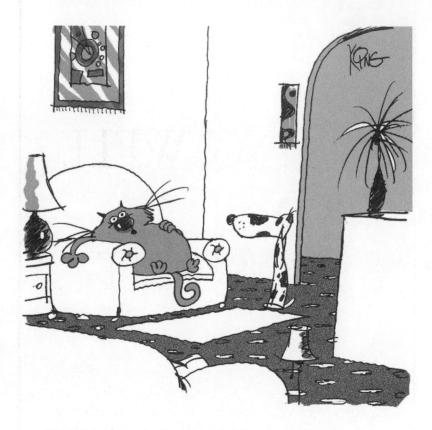

"My first three lives are for eating junk food and being lazy. My last six are for dieting and exercise."

Reprinted by permission of Jerry King.

2

EATING WELL AND STAYING FIT

Trials, temptations, disappointments—all these are helps instead of hindrances, if one uses them rightly. They not only test the fiber of character but strengthen it. Every conquering temptation represents a new fund of moral energy. Every trial endured and weathered in the right spirit makes a soul nobler and stronger than it was before.

James Buckham

No Pizza? No Problem!

Bad habits are like a comfortable bed, easy to get into, but hard to get out of.

Author Unknown

About a year ago, I was leaving a tiki hut in the East Village of New York City (bet you didn't know that NYC had tiki huts!) with two of my good (and very petite) friends when a random stranger shouted out, "Hey Blondie! You have a fat a**!"

Perhaps it was the two giant margaritas I had just imbibed, or maybe it was because this attack hit on the very core of a lifelong insecurity, but I immediately crumbled into a cocoon of tears.

My friends, of course, tried to console me, telling me he had meant "phat" not "fat" and that he was only a drunken stranger. But I had hit rock bottom, and I knew things, from that moment forth, had to change.

I was never "fat" per se, but I had been rather plump since I was a little girl. Blame it on growing up in a Jewish family with a very attentive grandma living across the street. Feeding was medicinal, and every day brought with it bagels, potatoes and an inordinate amount of sugar. After-school snacks of bialys or potato soup with some hot, fresh Jewish rye were the staple for me. I loved that time, and the food was a big part of it. "Eat! Eat!" To not eat would assuredly convince her that something was desperately wrong and cause endless concern. So I ate.

That night, as I sat there hating the phantom wino, the world and even myself, my friend gave me some good advice: Rather than indulging in yet another cycle of self-pity, do something about it. She had been seeing a nutritionist for years and was herself attempting the South Beach Diet. She recommended I give it a try.

In my mind, the South Beach Diet and other "low-carb" plans were all the same, and I was one of the masses who called them dangerous fads. I'd sit around with my friends, talking about how low-carb diets were dumb because as soon as you start eating "normal" again, you gain the weight back. I was sure South Beach wouldn't work, and it would be just another crazy waste of time.

Being the adventurous soul that I am though, I gave it a try. Phase 1, as we people in the plan call it, is very low-carbohydrate: no bread, no pasta, no sugar, no fruit or starch of any kind. Alcohol is a total no-no as well. Lean meats are your friends, fatty beefs and cheeses aren't.

But the overall plan is not low-carb, or even necessarily low-fat or low-calorie. It's more a modified lifestyle that teaches you to eat the right carbs, the right fats and the right proteins—and make it a part of your permanent life plan rather than a crash course into fitting into those too-tight jeans.

As a sugar aficionado, those first few days were a bit intense for me. I felt like I was in a state of perpetual PMS. I wasn't hungry; I ate my fill of egg whites and fresh veggies and grilled chicken—but what I was going through was hardcore sugar withdrawal. I'm a Sagittarius and thus possess a soul that demands instant gratification. And while my egg-white omelet with mozzarella and mushrooms was very satisfying, darn it, I was used to my morning bagel!

As those initial few days passed, I gradually grew less cranky. I ended up losing ten pounds, and an entire size, in the first two weeks.

The purpose of Phase 1 is a pseudo-detox; you are ridding your body of its addiction to sugar and simple carbs so that you can "retrain" it with the right ones later on. Once that hardcore phase is over, Phase 2 begins. During that phase, you gradually reintroduce your body to starches and fruits, very carefully and slowly, paying careful attention to what particular starches make your metabolism freak out. Refined sugars and starches are naughty now and always. Whole grains, oats, brown rice and sweet potatoes are all fine, and actually, pretty darn good for you if you don't go crazy with them.

South Beach is meant to be a lifestyle, not a diet, so of course, treats will happen. If it's your birthday, have the cake (a slice, not the entire sheet!), or indulge in a night of yummy Tex-Mex sometimes, as I do. The idea, though, is to not use those treats as a crutch. "Oh my God! I ate a brownie! It's all over . . . I might as well give up."

Over the course of about eight months, I lost fifty pounds and went from a size XL Misses to XS Juniors. I have more energy than I have ever had before, and I've learned to not only crave the good stuff but be repelled by that which is naughty. Do I cheat sometimes? Sure. It's called living. But I don't let food control me anymore. I'm too busy enjoying life on the Beach . . . which, every now and then, just might include a fresh, hot slice of seeded Jewish rye.

Aly Walansky

Morning Walk

It doesn't matter who my father was; it matters who I remember he was.

Anne Sexton

I am my father's daughter.

It was 6:30 on a Saturday morning and most sane people were still dreaming dreams, turning over in their warm beds and ignoring alarm clocks. Why was I walking around our neighborhood?

I am my father's daughter.

I thought about taking a shortcut—if I turned right at the next street, I could cut ten minutes off my walk and soon be home, savoring a warm cup of coffee with the morning paper.

I am my father's daughter.

This phrase became a mantra as I forced myself to walk those extra blocks. Ever since I had made the decision to lose weight by becoming more physically active, I had to daily talk myself out of excuses for not following through with my new exercise plan.

I am my father's daughter.

My father had been a smoker. He started smoking cigarettes when he was thirteen years old, stubbornly maintaining his habit into his seventies. My sister and I had
spent years trying to convince him to quit, but it took an
X-ray of his lungs to give him the incentive he needed to
finally do it, cold turkey, by sheer willpower. It had been
five years since he smoked a cigarette, and I was so proud
of him.

I am my father's daughter.

I was skinny as a teenager. Everyone was always
encouraging me to take seconds, and sometimes even
thirds, as a child. So I had gotten used to heaping my plate
full and then eating every single bite so that I didn't waste
any food. This was never a problem when I was thirteen
years old, but when I reached my thirties, the pounds
started adding up until the morning that I stepped on a
scale and realized that I was 255 pounds.

I am my father's daughter.

For a few years, I tried to find excuses. It was my
metabolism. I ate the same way I had always eaten, so
why else was I fat? Maybe I had a thyroid problem. As
more years passed and I moved into my forties, I blamed
the media for promoting a "thin culture" of unrealistic
body shapes. I scoffed at friends on fad diets, convincing
myself that my diet was healthier than theirs. I used to
laugh about my sister-in-law's skin turning orange from
eating too many carrots. Surely, a few extra pounds were
preferable to that?

I am my father's daughter.

When my doctor diagnosed me with high blood pressure and prescribed medication, he told me that if I lost
weight, I probably wouldn't need the medication. When I
fell down some stairs at work and the clinic x-rayed my
knee, I was told that the fall had not injured my knee but
that my knee didn't look good, due to the strain of my

weight. I decided I needed to make a change in my lifestyle.

I am my father's daughter.

After six months of half-hour walks, four to five times a week, I lost forty pounds. Then I added weight circuit training three times a week and monitored the portions of food on my plate, and now, almost two years later, I am seventy-five pounds lighter. At a recent family get-together to celebrate my father's five-year anniversary of giving up smoking, relatives exclaimed over my trimmer, fitter figure and asked me how I did it. I caught my dad's eye.

I am my father's daughter.

Deborah P. Kolodji

Gone to the Dogs

My doctor told me to stop having intimate dinners for four. Unless there are three other people.

Orson Welles

I've struggled with weight problems all my life.

During college, I tried every fad diet out there, from grapefruit juice with every meal to two weeks of nothing but boiled rice and fruit. From the time I was nineteen until I turned forty, my weight yo-yoed by as much as sixty pounds. I'd keep it off for a year or two, and then gradually the needle on the bathroom scale would creep back up.

Then a personal miracle entered my life, in the form of two Labrador retrievers.

My wife and I had been married for about a year when we got our second dog. Harley, our chocolate Lab, had just turned eight months when her sister, Buffy, a yellow Lab, was born. On that day, our lives changed forever.

All dogs require regular exercise to stay fit, but anyone who has ever owned a Labrador knows that it's a breed with boundless energy. Most experts agree a Lab needs at least two miles of brisk walking each day, and a typical Lab can do that and then be ready for a few hours of swimming or running afterward.

Harley and Buffy are no exception to the rule. We soon discovered that if we didn't give them a good workout each day, all their pent-up energy would lead them into all sorts of trouble around the house. As soon as Buffy was old enough, we instituted a regular exercise program for them, designed to tire them out so they'd sleep all night.

Weekdays begin at 6:00 AM with a brisk, half-mile to mile walk, depending on the weather. Only the heaviest snows or rains keep us from our morning constitutional. Then, after work, we do a minimum of two miles, often accompanied by games of chase-the-ball or stick. In the warm weather, we will often increase it to three miles.

But it doesn't end there. On the weekends the afternoon walk begins earlier, and usually involves a nice three- or four-mile hike in one of the local state parks.

Harley and Buffy are now eight and seven, respectively, and their exercise program, combined with nutritious food and no table scraps, has them in better shape than "any other Lab I've seen," according to our veterinarian.

The dogs love their daily exercise; the same can't be said for their masters. It's never easy to drag yourself from a warm bed on a cold or rainy winter day, bundle up, drive to the park and then trudge through the muck and puddles while a frenetic eighty-pound Energizer Bunny romps alongside you.

Even in the summer, there are often other things we'd rather be doing: relaxing after a hard day's work, taking care of the house, visiting friends. But when you make a commitment to a pet, it has to be honored. So we still take those walks, every day.

Of course, there's another reason we strap on those leashes.

Since dedicating ourselves to keeping our dogs fit, my wife and I have each lost more than forty pounds and kept it off. As soon as we realized the daily exercise was working as good for us as for our canine companions, we found the motivation we'd been lacking to stick to our own healthy diets.

Gone are the days when we'd give in to temptation and eat fast food, or buy popcorn and candy at the movies. In the past four years, I've had approximately twelve cans of soda. Before that, I drank it with lunch and dinner every day.

When we want Chinese food, we chop vegetables and tofu and make our own stir-fry. We measure portions of pasta and rice. The only snacks after dinner are fruit and sugar-free Jell-O. We've eliminated cheese on hamburgers and substituted veggie burgers for the beef patties.

On the occasions when we go out for dinner with friends or family, we make sure to fill up at the salad bar, skip the appetizers and order grilled chicken or some other healthy choice.

When one of us is lured into temptation, the other is always there to provide that most effective of all dissuasions: "Honey, if we eat that we'll have to walk an extra mile every day this week." Those words have the power to make either of us drop the candy or frozen pizza as if it were poison.

Of course, walking by itself isn't enough of an exercise program for a middle-aged person fighting the never-ending battle of the bulge. We've set up a small exercise room in our basement, with stationary bike, treadmill, elliptical machine and even a Bowflex for the arms and chest. On days when the rain, snow or temperature are too horrid for even diehard dog-walkers to venture outside, the home gym is a warm, dry alternative.

I've also gotten my wife to play golf with me, and we're

both bad enough at the game that we get plenty of exercise walking from cart to ball and back again.

But in the end, it all comes down to the dogs. They're our impetus for rising early each morning and heading back out again in the afternoons when all we want to do is sit on the deck with a glass of wine.

The funny thing is that all the excuses we had for never doing something like this before have turned out to be just that—excuses. No time? We still get everything done that we always did. It's too cold? Five minutes after coming home, it's like we never went out. Skipping a day won't hurt? Not only do Harley and Buffy make us crazy by bouncing off the walls, but we've found that we don't feel good if we skip a day.

Most importantly, all four of us are healthy, which means we'll be together for many years to come.

Greg Faherty

Skinny Munchies

Just think of all those women on the Titanic *who said, "No, thank you," to dessert that night. And for what!*

Erma Bombeck

Dieting is an embarrassing occupation, one I would really rather keep quiet about. My logic goes something like this: If no one sees me buying diet food, they certainly won't notice the extra fifty pounds I'm hauling around on my 5'3" frame. Perhaps it isn't the diet that's as embarrassing as the failure to stay on the diet.

Discretion is essential when shopping, and knowing your way around the local grocery store is crucial. It's reassuring to know where the Marshmallow Mateys are when you're in a hurry for a nutritious breakfast. Or which aisle to avoid when toting a toddler with a long reach. Or where along the cookie aisle some teenage bag boy has stocked the Chips Ahoy.

After moving to a small town from a large metropolitan city, I was unable to locate a favorite low-cal snack in the local grocery store, so I decided to inquire at the register.

Right away, a voice inside my head raised an alarm. *Don't do that,* the voice warned. *Just keep looking. It might be embarrassing if you ask and they don't have it.*

Oh, give me a break, I argued with myself, *I'm thirty years old. I can certainly ask for a product in a grocery store. I am an adult.*

You really might want to think this through a bit more, dear, the voice wheedled.

Bug off, I answered.

At least I wasn't talking out loud like the lady two aisles over debating whether Windex would kill the ants in her petunia bed.

At the checkout, a slim, young woman whose name badge read "Clarista" began checking out my groceries. I got my nerve up and leaned over the package of Ding-Dongs just crossing her scanner.

"Do you know if you carry Skinny Munchies?" I inquired.

Pausing in midscan, she replied, "Skinny what?" A tiny smile spread across her face.

"Skinny Munchies," I answered, lowering my eyes in a flicker of panic. "They're a Weight Watchers product, uh, little chips that are legal for Weight Watchers to, uh, snack on . . ."

"Oh, that's the cutest thing I've ever heard!" she exclaimed, breaking into a big grin and reaching for the large microphone stretched across her cash register. "Mr. Sidensticker," she called with delight, "do you know if we sell something called Skinny Munchies?"

Mr. Sidensticker, the store manager stationed in the customer service booth one aisle away, reached for his microphone. "Skinny what?" he asked.

"Skinny Munchies," she answered over the PA system, ignoring my stammered pleas to "never mind."

"She says they're a Weight Watchers product. Isn't that cute?"

"Never heard of 'em," Mr. Sidensticker's voice boomed back. "Do they work?"

Feeling the amusement of every well-proportioned shopper standing in line behind me, I managed to choke out, "No, uh, uh, no, never mind . . . it's not important." Desperate for a quick exit, I grabbed my Cheez Doodles and Diet Orange Crush and began pulling them over the scanner myself.

"I don't know, I'll ask her," Clarista's voice echoed. Still holding down the "on" button of the microphone, she turned to interrogate me further, "Do they work?"

Shoppers throughout the store looked up to the speakers in the ceiling, anxiously awaiting an answer. Sucking in my stomach and pitching my Cini-Minis down the conveyer belt, I offered breathlessly, "Well, that's obvious, isn't it?" Rushing to scrawl out a check, I made my escape.

Never again would I argue with the smug voice that was smiling in my head and tut-tutting, *I told you so!* From now on, if I can't find the diet product I'm looking for in the grocery store, I'll save myself a grocery-cart-full of embarrassment and substitute a high-calorie equivalent.

Sally Clark

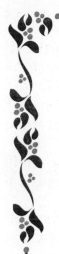

Amazing Apple Vinaigrette

MAKES 2 SERVINGS
EACH SERVING: 0 GRAMS SATURATED FAT

1 handful of fresh parsley
¼ cup flaxseed oil
½ cup unsweetened applesauce
¼ cup apple juice
1 tablespoon brown sugar
¼ cup apple cider vinegar
2 garlic cloves, chopped
¼ teaspoon salt

Toss all ingredients into a blender or food processor and puree until smooth and creamy. Serve with mixed greens.

Note: You can store this vinaigrette in a covered container in the refrigerator for up to two days.

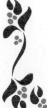

Reprinted from The Gold Coast Cure. ©2005 *Andrew Larson, M.D., Ivy Ingram Larson. Health Communications, Inc.*

Trading Fat Cells for Barbells

To be tested is good. The challenged life may be the best therapist.

Gail Sheehy

She whips out her appointment book and cheerfully rattles off open times. "First thing in the morning is always good," she lies.

Nothing is good first thing in the morning except coffee in bed. In fact, the best thing first thing in the morning IS my bed.

"What about 5:00 or 10:00 AM?" Dancing brown eyes shimmer over a smile that cuts her face in half. She is all teeth and joy. Even her name is cheerful—Lorri Ann. I had hoped for someone as somber about this situation as I. If fitness centers are great places to meet people, I wanted someone I could relate to right off the bat. Someone who knows that this is the last stop on the road to the end of the world. At least the world as I knew it.

"Weight training is so exciting. You won't believe how it will make you feel. We can reshape your body like PLAY-

DOH. When you come in, first thing we'll do is fat testing. Then we'll measure your dimensions."

I was never keen on tests in school. My fat did not wiggle for joy upon notice that it too would endure a test of its own.

Her enthusiasm ricocheted off a forty-foot ceiling. "You're really gonna love it," she lied again.

Cautiously, I returned to the gigantic lobby of the big, fancy health facility (BFHF) early one Friday. Thawing out under the bright lights of the BFHF, I pondered the lighting. Brightness burst through big windows and down from the ceiling like those merciless bulbs in dressing rooms that highlight your figure flaws when you are at your most vulnerable—trying on clothes.

"I'm so glad you're here, Suzan!" Lorri Ann Code bounced toward me with that beaming face of hers.

Health clubs make me feel uneasy. Over the years I have entered their doors after occasional bouts of bottoming out from my lifestyle of denial, indulgence, denial, indulgence, repeat. These clubs attract spandex-laden lassies with perky ponytails who strut in glittery tights. I wear old maternity pants just to get through the buffet line during the holidays.

"Let's begin!"

I filled out health history forms, then, with Lorri Ann, established "measurable goals." It was important that I understand what I wanted out of this undertaking.

I wanted it to be over.

I also wanted stronger bones and tighter everything else. I knew that New Year's resolutions often fail because we promise on the heads of our children to give up something without considering that we are actually taking on a lifestyle change. Clearly, bowing out of this commitment would be difficult with Captain Code around. Accountability this time had a face with a big grin on it.

We headed for the equipment—gigantic contraptions of metal with pulleys and cables connected to an array of weights. Captain Code demonstrated each apparatus, which strengthen and tone different muscles. I followed her lead, receiving encouraging remarks and gentle corrections, "Keep your wrists straight, put your head back, align your back, don't rotate your shoulders." She wrote copious notes on my workout sheet denoting the number of repetitions, weight used, posture, seat height, where my feet belonged and so forth.

Code does not tolerate a sloppy performance. "You'll get great benefits but you have to use the machines correctly. When you come back next time, you'll go first and I'll tell you what you are doing right and what you are doing wrong. It's the best way to learn."

I can hardly believe I am finally keeping a promise I'd made for fifteen years—to learn weight training.

"The first four weeks we build a base," she says. "After that, we'll develop a program where you can work your upper body one day, lower another or do a combination. Does it hurt yet?" she smiles. "Four more, three, two, one, rest and stretch for sixty seconds. Do you mind being sore in the morning? Wait until tomorrow night!"

I claim I don't mind pain later, but in the heat of the moment I am adverse to it. She says something else but I don't hear it, distracted by a man with arms the size of the Sierra Nevada mountains. The next fifteen reps whip by. Some views in the BFHF are not designed to go unnoticed. People of all ages and sizes are there. A variety of "before, during and afters," I consider. It is comforting to see folks in their thirties, forties and fifties. I thought mostly twenty-year-old blondes in tights went to health clubs. At forty-five, I was in the right demographic in my Big Dog gym pants.

We concluded with a cardiovascular workout. Captain

Code gave me a choice of stair steppers, exercise bikes, treadmills and other pieces of equipment designed with your sweat in mind. "You'll start to burn fat after twenty minutes."

"Put the timer on thirty," I bravely retort.

"Good girl! You're doing great!" she says this for the twentieth time. I love hearing it. An hour of being the center of attention when I am used to ignoring my needs in lieu of family demands felt surprisingly rejuvenating. I wanted more.

Lorri Ann whipped out a set of headphones called "Cardio-Theater" and plugged them into a box on the machine. Two television sets hang from the ceiling in front of us. "This TV is Channel 4, that one is Channel 15, or you can listen to music or talk shows."

Working out wasn't so bad after all. The handle of my treadmill measured my heart rate. I felt sudden exhilaration. I had a trainer! At long last I was learning the correct way to use intimidating equipment that would tone my body in new and unexpected ways. And perhaps my attitude might get toned in the process. For the first time in ages, I felt like a star.

Suzan Davis

The Exchange Rate

After years of inactivity, my expanding waistline forced me to swap vegetables. I traded my membership in the couch potato club for one in a squash club.

After handing over my credit card for initiation and monthly dues, I discovered fitness didn't come cheap. With the money I had left, I bought a squash racket and a tennis dress that fit my budget better than my body. It groaned when I zipped it up, but if I didn't breathe too deeply maybe the seams would hold until I lost ten pounds.

Over the next few months, between running around the court to pick up missed balls and the odd rally where I actually returned the shot, my outfit stopped protesting. It took another couple of months for the court, which rivaled a football field in size, to shrink to standard dimensions. The rallies lengthened as balls that had previously whizzed past my racquet were now within reach. Having previously exchanged vegetables, I now exchanged vowels as I moved from fat to fit. The time had come to ratchet up my exercise program another notch. Although the club director had mentioned a workout room on the top floor, for the first six months I hadn't had the energy to make it past the second floor. Now I was ready.

The third floor housed two small rooms, divided by a wall of mirrors, to form one larger area. Stationary bicycles and rowing machines filled one side; the other held racks of free weights. Large doorways allowed a banked wooden track to circle the perimeter of the two rooms.

I headed for the track, sprinted off and promptly collided with a runner charging through the doorway. He pointed to a sign and continued running. I hobbled over to read the sign, which directed members to run clockwise on even days of the month and counterclockwise on odd days to avoid uneven build-up of muscles. I pictured a clock, complete with hands, and set out again in the opposite direction.

Off to an inauspicious start, I figured my running experience could only improve. With eight laps to the mile, the hardest part would be keeping track of the number. I needn't have worried. By the end of my first lap, I was huffing and puffing so hard I had to stop. Something was very wrong.

Stumbling off the track, I realized the "something" was "someone." Me. The flushed, sweat- and mascara-streaked face that greeted me in the multiple mirrors confirmed it. I erased the word "fit" from my vocabulary and replaced it with "cardiac victim."

After my heart stopped pounding, I crept downstairs to the women's locker room and splashed cold water on my face. As the redness faded, I made a vow to my reflection: one day I would run a mile, if not with ease and grace, at least without sounding like a steam engine. And I'd wear waterproof mascara so I wouldn't look like a raccoon at the finish line.

Over the next few months, I arrived at the club an hour before my squash game and forced myself upstairs to the track. I ran clockwise and huffed. I ran counterclockwise and puffed. After being rear-ended when I slowed suddenly, I learned to keep to the outside of the track in the "slow" lane when another pair of feet pounded behind me. I considered slapping a bumper sticker on my rear end that said "Beginner Runner—Beware" but decided anyone close enough to read the sticker was about to crash into me anyway.

I used a clicker to record the laps. Not that I couldn't count, but it made me feel more like a real runner. Although my laps started adding up, they still didn't total the magic number eight. I kept at it. Two months passed and I spent more time running and less time huffing and puffing. Other runners stopped offering to drive me to the emergency room of the nearest hospital.

Then came the day I stopped thinking and simply ran, feet pounding and arms pumping at my sides. Just me and the track. The laps glided by until I glanced at the clicker in my hand and saw the counter change to seven. Only one more lap stood between me and my goal. I ran on.

I rounded the last turn, crossed the finish line and stopped in amazement, nearly knocking down the guy behind me. I apologized and hastily stepped off the track to savor my victory. I had done it. I had metamorphosed from couch potato to Queen of the Track. Okay, maybe just her lady-in-waiting.

Having conquered the mile, I've set new goals. I've started training for two miles. Next I'll go for three miles. Then four miles. Then marathons—though at the rate I'm going, I'll probably be running in the geriatric category. I don't care. I am runner—hear me roar!

Harriet Cooper

Facing the Lady in the Mirror

Fitness—if it came in a bottle, everybody would have a great body.

Cher

Pudgy, never quite good enough—that's what the lady looking back at me from the mirror preached. I swallowed all of it.

My daughter's Christmas present changed everything. It looked innocent enough: a few printed lines in an envelope. But my stomach turned inside out as I read them—a gift certificate for twenty-four fitness classes. My daughter smiled expectantly. I smiled back through clenched teeth.

That night, the lady in the mirror yelled at me. "Ignore the gift," she said. "You can't display your pudgy body at the gym."

January came; the lady in the mirror convinced me to do nothing. February rolled around; she won again, and the guilt grew. March arrived; another round with my nemesis ended up in a screaming match. By the time April came, I stood up to her, for my daughter's sake; I'd find a way to survive the humiliation. But she smiled wickedly. I stalled once more.

Out of excuses and scared to death, I eventually entered the dreaded fitness center on a Monday in May, wearing an oversized T-shirt and baggy sweatpants. The young girl at the desk was a size 2 at the most—she probably never ate a cookie in her life. She pointed to the aerobics room.

When I walked in, the lady in the mirror stared back at me. Who let her in? The entire front wall was one huge mirror, top to bottom, left to right! No place to hide. My pudgy arms, jiggly thighs and enormous buns looked back at me. I had to get out of there.

But just as I made my move to the door, the music started and the crowded room came into order. I was shoved into place. The instructor said the aerobic segment would last thirty-five minutes. Thirty-five little minutes— maybe I could survive them.

I did my best to move to the motivational music. The singer told me I looked good today, but she was lying. Ask the lady in the mirror, she'll tell you. While the singer told me to give it my all, I cheated every place I could. I prayed no one would notice my smaller steps and heavy breathing. The lady in the mirror laughed. Then, the long thirty-five minutes were over.

I went home and had an ice cream sundae with an extra cherry on top.

Wednesday came around too fast, and the lady in the mirror convinced me to skip the aerobics class. I grabbed my favorite magazine, a candy bar and plopped myself on the couch. That's when the phone rang. "You remember you have class today, Mom?"

I dragged my still sore body to the fitness center. The same size 2 girl sat at the front desk, and the same wall-to-wall mirror glared at me. The dreaded class started. Ten minutes into it, my skin dripped with sweat, and my nose screamed for me to get away from my own smelly self. But as I concentrated on the moves, my body woke me up from the inside out. The awkwardness left, and I enjoyed myself just a little bit.

After class, I bought a new pair of workout pants, the kind the other ladies wore. And I splurged for a red water bottle—if I was going to make it through the twenty-four classes, I'd do it in style! Take that, lady in the mirror!

Friday was rainy, and the lady in the mirror said to take it easy. But my new pants and water bottle called out to me. I went to class and survived. Three lessons under my belt! "Twenty-one to go!" the lady in the mirror scoffed.

When I got home, my daughter had left a little card waiting for me on the kitchen table. "One whole week done, Mom! Way to go." This time, the lady in the mirror cringed as I smiled.

The awareness of my body snowballed into all of my life. I became more conscious of what I ate. I found myself choosing a few carrots instead of a candy bar. I drank water with lemon instead of that sugary soda. I made up a new dessert with baked apples and sugar-free Jell-O.

Twelve classes down the road, I was having fun, not needing to cheat quite as much anymore. One of the ladies said I looked smaller. I stepped on the scale when I got home—three pounds off! I wouldn't boast to the lady in the mirror yet, but I smiled all evening and skipped dessert.

Over the weekend, at my son's cross-country meet, I ran from one point to another to catch him on the trail. I noticed I didn't run out of breath. Was I really getting fit? I decided I would try to run one whole mile at home the next Saturday.

"Who are you kidding?" the lady in the mirror said.

When Saturday came around, I laced my shoes, ignoring the lady in the mirror's laughter. I started to run; one whole mile later, I stopped, my heart soaring. The lady in the mirror didn't dare talk to me again that day.

My jeans got a bit too loose. I had fun buying a new pair. To celebrate, I went for another run; this time, I made it through the two-mile marker. Could I do three? That would be next week's challenge.

With the twenty-four classes up, I signed up for another session. The numbers on the scale kept creeping down, ever so slowly. I ran each Saturday, pushing a bit farther each week. Me, the pudgy lady, running five miles! By now I found an almost permanent smile in my heart.

A year later and fifteen pounds lighter, I was loving every class, hardly ever missing a day. I moved from the back row to the front and even looked in the mirror occasionally. The lady staring back at me didn't look too angry anymore. And most important, she had stopped telling me how ugly I was. At times she almost smiled.

My aerobics teacher got pregnant and taught through much of the pregnancy. At about her sixth month, she asked me to stay after class. When all the ladies were gone, she brought up the idea of me taking over her class.

The lady in the mirror stood up in a fury, back to her old tricks.

"I can't," I said. "I'm just a bit too pudgy, if you know what I mean . . ." She gave me a puzzled look.

"Would you at least give it a try? I'd teach you all you need to know until you can be certified," the instructor persisted.

I dreamed on the way home, but the lady in the mirror turned mean, laughing out loud. I knew then that the confrontation was inescapable.

When home, I slowly walked up to the mirror, mentally preparing myself for the showdown. The lady in the mirror knew I couldn't do without her. She had been my comfortable enemy, my safe escape from life. Would I survive the dare?

Taking a deep breath, I squared my body and braced myself to defend my newfound self. I opened my eyes to stare her down.

She just stood there, perfectly quiet.

I took a long, long look at her. She wasn't the way I remembered her: the lady gazing back at me had a new air of confidence about her. I liked her; she looked lovely.

I burst out crying. She cried with me.

I filled out the application and was hired soon after. Since then, I have been certified as a group exercise instructor, and I teach fitness classes, daring women from all walks of life to stare down the lady in the mirror at first—and then to make her a best friend.

And we are winning, one mirror at a time.

Barbara A. Croce

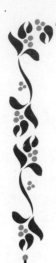

Greek Rice

MAKES ABOUT 6 CUPS
EACH ⅓ CUP: 4 GRAMS PROTEIN, 15 GRAMS CARBOHYDRATE

2 tablespoons pure-pressed extra virgin olive oil
1 diced small yellow onion
1 minced garlic clove
1½ cups long-grain brown rice, rinsed and drained
3 cups low-sodium chicken stock or 3 cups water
3 tablespoons fresh lemon juice
2 teaspoons dried oregano
⅓ cup diced Kalamata olives
⅓ cup minced fresh parsley
freshly ground black pepper to taste
½ cup crumbled feta cheese

In a medium saucepan with a tight-fitting lid, heat oil over medium-high heat. When oil is hot, add onion and garlic and sauté until softened, about 5 minutes. Add rice and sauté 2 minutes, stirring occasionally. Add stock or water. Bring to a boil.

Cover and reduce heat to low. Simmer 45 to 50 minutes. Remove from heat and let sit, covered and undisturbed, for 10 minutes. Remove lid and fluff rice with a fork. Add lemon juice, oregano, Kalamata olives, parsley and black pepper. Stir in feta cheese and mix well. Taste, and adjust seasonings.

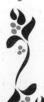

Reprinted from The Schwarzbein Principle Cookbook. ©1999
*Diana Schwarzbein, M.D., Nancy Deville and Evelyn Jacob. Health
Communications, Inc*

A Diet for Life—Literally

The first wealth is health.

Emerson

My mother is a fighter. A fighter who was diagnosed with breast cancer at the age of forty-eight and then diagnosed a second time with terminal liver cancer at fifty-two. The first time around had been rough—surgeries to literally cut out the cancer-ridden cells, chemotherapy that ravaged her petite body, and medicines that manipulated her moods and left her feeling sick and weak.

When she found out four years later that the cancer had returned, and much worse than before, she decided to take a different approach. Since it was impossible to remove the cancer surgically, she set about to transform her body from the inside out. This meant enlisting the help of an "alternative therapies" doctor, someone who would coach her on the path to recovery through mind, body and spirit.

Always an active and healthy individual, my mother was shocked the day that her doctor sat her down and began to rattle off the dramatic dietary changes that she would need to make during her treatment. No meat, no eggs, no dairy, no sugar . . . the list went on and on. At the time, the diet was not merely a suggestion or option, it was my mother's livelihood, and so although it seemed a bit drastic to all of us, we encouraged and aided her from the very first day. Her new diet consisted of hearty meals that were restricted to organic whole grains, vegetables and the occasional piece of fruit or white seafood.

None of us had anticipated the impact that my mother's diet would have on our lives. Gone were the evenings when we would come home to the delicious smells of freshly baked cookies wafting through the air. Instead, we found dinners of brightly colored steamed veggies (embarrassingly, some were unrecognizable to our meat-and-potato palates), organic brown rice and whole-grain breads with hummus and olive oil. We had known that this would be a huge task for our mother but never considered (or imagined) how greatly her new eating habits would affect the rest of the family. Needless to say, my initial reaction urged me to grab take-out more than once on drives home from work.

Yet over the course of a couple of months, our family became accustomed to steamed instead of fried foods, bright foods instead of boxed foods. We developed a taste for those unpronounceable vegetables, especially when we added a bit of olive oil and garlic and sautéed them. In fact, they tasted even better than they had before, when they were drenched in salt and butter.

We spent more time on the patio, grilling fresh fish with vegetable kabobs, enjoying the warm summer breeze. We created our own organic garden in the backyard, tending to the tiny plants until they grew strong enough to produce ripe foods, perfect for spring salads and fulfilling in a way that only homegrown goods can be. We started an herb garden and then taught ourselves how to use the fresh sprigs to bring out natural flavors without heavy calories.

Without chocolaty sweets strewn about, fresh fruit Popsicles became indulgent treats. A plump orange or tangerine satisfied a semisweet tooth. And even the worst of late-night cravings was nothing that a sliced apple and yogurt for dipping couldn't quench.

We began regularly taking the vitamins and supplements that our bodies were deficient in, fueling ourselves the right way. Late-night strolls became commonplace, and Libby, the family dog, finally received the long daily walks that she deserved.

Most importantly, we saw our mother become stronger, happier and healthier. The rest of us shed the extra pounds that had been lingering in unpleasant places and felt our bodies grow leaner every day. A renewed sense of spirit and self took over each one of us, and its dazzling positive energy filled our home.

Four months after her second diagnosis, my mother's "alternative" doctor called. There was news, and whether it was good or bad none of us knew. The week before she had gone in for a complete body scan that would reveal any other spots that the cancer had quietly crept into. We all spent that night awake, lying in bed in silent prayer. How much longer would we have with this woman who was so eager to take on life full-force when most would give in and give up? Another year? Another month?

The next morning a smile played on the doctor's lips as he sat my mother down and told her that the traces of cancer had vanished. It had left her body; leaving only minimal scarring in the areas it had once inhabited. Her body was healthy—on the inside as well as the outside.

Celebration was in order—a feast of all the wonderful foods we had grown to love. Although the cancer was gone, there would be no chancing it with chocolate cake relapses and soft, chewy candy. We had given her body the best shot that it had—a healthy, fresh and natural diet, full of the good things that Mother Nature intended to nourish us.

It took a strong family and a strong heart to take on an entirely new diet with such ambition and eagerness. It took driving a few miles out of the way to find a natural grocery store with organic produce, and a few extra dollars to buy the fresh stuff instead of what was prepackaged or boxed. It took a bit of determination to get off the couch, flip off the TV, and head outside for sunshine and exercise. Yet the change that it made in my life, my mother's and my family's is undeniable. My mother continues to do well. She still undergoes the medical preventative treatments while maintaining her alternative life changes, and no cancer has returned thus far.

I won't say that I never get a sudden urge for sweets (or that I never indulge just a tiny bit), but I realize now how amazing the human body is and to give it any less than the wholesome things it deserves is truly only cheating yourself.

Jessica Blaire

A Skinny By-Product

*I bought a talking refrigerator that said "Oink"
every time I opened the door. It made me hungry
for pork chops.*

Marie Mott

Dr. Choi is a wonderful doctor, but she says bad things.
Two of her words punched me in the repository of my ill-
conceived eating habits. "Cholesterol" and "pre-diabetes"
aren't exactly the reassuring words that I wanted to hear.
They deflated my feeling of invincibility.

The day that she delivered the cholesterol message, she
had another word that I wouldn't vote for. She said "oatmeal." I said "raisin bran." She said "oatmeal." I said
"shredded wheat." She said "oatmeal." I said "Wheatina."
She said "oatmeal." My grasping response to her final reit-
eration of the oatmeal decree was "but oatmeal has the
consistency of snot." With that said I went home with a
variety pack of wallpaper paste, better known as oatmeal.
I eventually settled on raisin, date and walnut and have
since come to like it. That meant the end of an English
muffin with a generous layer of butter, a mountain of

peanut butter and a pool of grape jelly. Breakfast was to be a new experience.

Had I not seen an almost instant weight loss, I would have returned to my gooey culinary wonderland. The day that Dr. Choi delivered the devastating cholesterol message, I weighed in at 228 pounds. A few months later my six-foot frame was carrying a mere 210 pounds. Surprisingly, I hadn't been hungry. The only change in my eating habits was my breakfast. Who would have thought that an English muffin with a few upgrades would weigh eighteen pounds?

This past February "pre-diabetes" was Dr. Choi's word for the day. I would have preferred "psoriasis" or even "pneumonia." As before she had a one-track mind and insisted on repeating pre-diabetes until it became part of my vocabulary. She set me up with a hospital lecture on the subject. I decided that I didn't know enough about this ailment to tamper with my diet until after the lecture. This stalling action gave me another three weeks of butter pecan ice cream floating knee-deep in maple syrup and one last apple pie—every piece topped with succulent vanilla ice cream.

On the first of March I held a funeral service for raw sugar and stocked up on my choice of sugar substitutes. I weighed myself on the day that sugar died, 208 lbs. The only other dietary change was switching from white bread to dark bread. Today is August 27 and I've weighed a mere 180 pounds for over a month. I didn't change the *quantity* that I eat; I only changed *what* I eat, and I'm not hungry.

My wife, Linda, jokingly referred to me as her "Chubby Hubby" until my ribs made a reappearance following a thirty-year absence. My cholesterol is under control, but the jury is still out on my pre-diabetic condition. Should that condition need further attention, I'll deal with my almost-daily potato chip and dry-roasted peanut habit. I realize that addressing health issues after the fact isn't the best way to eat. For now, however, I'm content to lose weight on the lousy diagnosis installment plan. Giving up one special food at a time is easier than trying to do them all at the same time. While my method is not approved by the American Medical Association, it seems to work better for me than any other technique that I've tried.

I've lost forty-eight pounds with simple changes that have nothing to do with starvation or fasting. This technique might not work for everyone, but it did wonders for me because I am, and always have been, a light eater. My problem was that since I discovered Snicker bars and high-octane Coke and Pepsi, I relied on multiple vitamins to balance my diet. One disease modification at a time, I'm getting back on track and becoming the healthy man that God intended me to be. A note of caution to stockholders in either Pringles or Planters corporations: your profit margins might be affected by this visit.

Ed VanDeMark

My Own Way

In the midst of movement and chaos, keep stillness inside of you.

Deepak Chopra

I am blessed with beautiful big eyes, a full mouth, long legs, soft hair and eyebrows that get compliments from every waxer I've been to. My breasts aren't large, but with the right bra they can be ample enough. My hips aren't slim, but they support me and held up my ten-pound baby when he was in the womb. My legs are no longer slender, but they are filled with muscle gained from daily walks and exercise. And then there's my stomach, my paunch as I call it, the bane of my existence, partly caused by my excessive sugar consumption, partly by heredity. I am beautiful, though, and sexy in my own way. I am athletic, but by no means a tiny woman. I am finding my way to peace with myself.

I began swimming when I was six years old. I took to it immediately and continued to compete until graduating high school. I was a record-breaker in my school and a state championship competitor. I loved every second of it. And then I graduated, and fear came into me about so many things in life. I was resisting every-thing and everyone. I was scared and angry at the world and, as usually happens, took it out more on myself than on others. One way I did this was by rob-bing myself of my innate pleasure of the water. I still taught swimming and coached for awhile, but I stuck to a complaint of shoulder injury and never swam again.

At first it was easy to maintain my body, but as I got older and life settled down and a baby was born, I lost who I was in many senses. I began exercising again. I focused mostly on walking, as long walks give me the solitude and quiet that enables my best thinking and allows me to work out things in my life. But I knew I needed more than just that. I listened to the media and popular views and took my cue from them.

First I tried yoga and later Pilates. I loved them both for the stretches that my body needed and the calming focus, but I just couldn't attach myself to them as some people do. I tried aerobic classes. I heard how they are great for getting your heart rate up and getting you into shape, so it had to be the right thing to do. But not for me. I felt like I was an awkward thirteen-year-old again, back at the school dance without a date. I have no rhythm, and no matter how long I stuck out the classes, I just felt like I was an enormously tall and lumbering she-male stomping across the back of the room. So I dropped that. Then I headed into the gym and tried the wonderful EFX machines (it's like cross-country skiing on a slope). I loved these. I stuck with it for almost a year and loved to feel the sweat pouring off and the knowledge that I was accomplishing something.

But as time went on, I felt like a hamster in a wheel. Round and round I'd go with ten televisions blasting me with images and music playing overhead and everyone else there looking tiny and cute with darling exercise clothes on looking at each other! I couldn't take it. I knew I was going to stop that as well. None of it was me. None of it fit, even though it was what was supposed to work. Everyone else seemed to be finding their thing, the thing that made them feel good, that they stuck to, that made them powerful. I wanted mine too, and I knew what it was.

One morning I got up and decided that this was it; I was headed back to the pool and no shoulder injury was going to stop me. If I had to, I would spend the entire time kicking. And in the beginning that's what I did. I kicked a lot, swam a little. Then swam some more. Then some more. Now I can't wait to get into that pool. I feel like I've come home. This is what works for me, for my body, for my personality, for my emotions. It's new to think of exercise in those terms, but it's true. We feel things when we move our bodies. The key is listening to those feelings and finding the thing that brings peace and power into your body.

I will never be a tiny woman, and I'm fine with that now, more fine with it than I've ever been before. My weight on the scale doesn't change much, but the tightening of my body is apparent to everyone. I feel strong. I feel capable. I feel powerful in my own skin. Through these feelings I can see and know my own beauty and sexiness. I am no longer forcing my body into positions or activities that feel just that—forced. I am going with the flow of what works for me. When I swim, I feel better, healthier and more proud of myself. That is what exercise needs to be about. Those feelings are what will keep you coming back, even on the days when you don't want to.

I experimented, tried things on and felt how they fit.

But as with everything in life, I had to listen to myself, listen to my own body; it tells me where it needs to be. When you find that place that feels right, stay there, love it, work in it, and allow the feelings of strength and power to be yours.

Colleen Kappeler

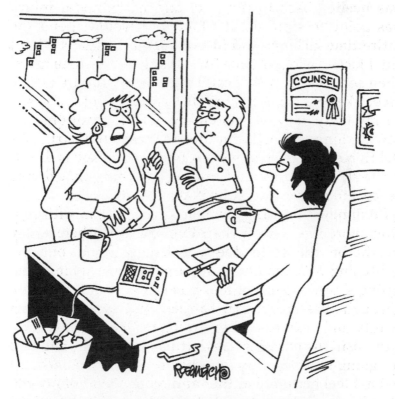

"He didn't exactly call me overweight, but he keeps trying to stick refrigerator magnets on me!"

Reprinted by permission of Dan Rosanditch.

Weight-Loss Wisdom
from a Toddler

Much may be learned about any society by studying the behavior and accepted ideas of its children.

Robertson Davies

It's no fun carrying around the "baby weight" as your child ages. I knew if I didn't make some changes soon I would still have those extra pounds when my son started school. But when I decided to lose thirty pounds, I didn't do it alone. I had help from meeting leaders, my husband and my own personal miniguru, the toddler. In my weight-loss journey, I found I learned a lot just by observing him.

My son doesn't use a stair-climber, lift weights or own a treadmill. He finds simpler ways to get the job done. He runs—an empty field or backyard is perfect. If he climbs stairs, they're real ones and not the kind found in a gym. The lesson: Use what you have. Go up and down the stairs at your local community center, museum or aquarium with your child. I guarantee you'll know you've worked out. That is, if you can get out of bed the next day. If your child has a favorite musical act (Wiggles or Laurie Berkner, anyone?) pop in a video and dance along. You'll eat up some of that vast supply of energy while you burn calories, and you'll both have fun doing it.

The other day, we rode our bikes as a family through our neighborhood and ended up at a local park, where we discovered a trail off the beaten track. My son took a minute to warm up to it, but once he did, he delighted in exploring. Despite our exhaustion from pedaling our bicycles in the Florida heat, his enthusiasm was contagious. We deviated from our plan and stayed awhile longer.

Lots of workout advice extols the virtues of mini-workouts. While the plan may be meant to allow busy parents a way to get a workout in, they also seem tailor-made for a youngster. I circuit train—kid-style. My son's program on a recent afternoon involved bouncing in his bounce house, traveling over to his wading pool for a few quick full-body splashes and then finishing off with laps around the backyard.

Something else I've learned from the little one is that a little bit of food goes a long way. My son will eat small portions of food and stop when he's full. Then, no matter how much you prod, plead or insist, not one more bite will pass through his lips. Not even if it's his absolute favorite food. He savors what he truly enjoys and doesn't bother finishing what doesn't appeal to him. He only eats when he's hungry—you can be sure he'll let you know when that happens! And he doesn't linger over meals; twenty-five minutes is a long time for him to spend eating. When he has finished, it's on to the next adventure.

My tiny mentor is always ready to try something new. Who knew he would enjoy food like avocados or cucumbers, or that the highlight of his day would be a bicycle ride? Getting out of a rut is good for all of us—adults and children alike. Sometimes you don't have to look very far to find a new perspective on diet and exercise. Just spend a little time with the child in your life for inspiration and motivation.

Tricia Finch

10 Tricks to Help You Stay on Your Diet

Tell everyone you know you are on a diet. Ask them to help you behave. Ask them to work with you, for instance, when choosing a restaurant or activity. There will be places where you will not find appropriate food on the menu, and this can help you avoid them. With a team supporting your effort, you will be more apt to stay on your diet. You will want to lose weight because you won't want to let them down or embarrass yourself.

Keep a chart. Post a chart in the bathroom on your mirror with all of your vital statistics: date, weight, and measurements of your chest, waist, hips, thighs and upper arms. Update it at the same time each week. If you are ALMOST a certain weight or size, write down the higher one to keep you on your path.

Set realistic goals. On your weight/measurement chart, write down your goals. How much is your ideal weight? What is the halfway point? What weight will you be when you've lost one-fourth of the target weight? Highlight the weeks when you reach these goals.

Reward yourself! When you reach each goal, give yourself a present. Buy something great, sized just a bit small. Make sure you love it so you'll want to fit into it. Hang it where you see it every single day. Keep trying it on. Do not wear it until it fits perfectly. The rewards will help keep you on the right track. And tell your support team about them, so when they see this reward, they'll know you are seeing success.

Learn how your body works and help it. If you know that soda stimulates your hunger, don't drink it, and by all means, get rid of any you have in the house. If you know that something fills you more than something else, take advantage of it. If you know you must be active, then be very active. Learn what makes your body tick, and help it tick faster.

Change how you look. Sometimes a new look can help your body feel weight-loss worthy. Change your hairstyle or hair color. When people notice the change, they will also see how much weight you have lost. It's natural for people to reward you with compliments. These compliments will keep you motivated. Having fabulous posture helps you look thinner and helps you tighten muscles. Slouching only makes you look round and fat and sloppy.

Keep a journal. Write down what you eat and when. Then when you see changes, you can analyze why you lost or did not lose weight. Write down how you feel from day to day. Were you tired? Did you feel energetic? Did you break your diet? Did you feel hunger? Did something happen to trigger a bad habit? Besides having a place to vent, it gives you something to do besides going into the kitchen to find something to eat.

Exercise a lot. You have heard this before, and if it were not true, it would not be mentioned as much. Exercise makes the weight come off faster, and it helps keep it off once you have lost it. Exercise can be as simple as turning the slow walk with your dog into a brisk walk with your dog.

Photograph yourself as you go. Post the pictures around your home so you and others can see where you were. A mirror is often deceiving, but pictures do not lie. Plus, you'll have a record of your hard work when you reach each goal, especially your final goal.

Flaunt it. Wiggle your stuff. Strut. Feel proud. Let the world know how good you feel by how you move your body.

Felice Prager

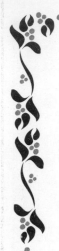

Raspberries & Cream Soy Smoothie

MAKES 2 SERVINGS
EACH SERVING: 0 GRAMS SATURATED FAT

1 cup soy milk or low-fat milk
8 ounces silken tofu (or ½ package of Nasoya
    Silken Tofu)
1½ cups frozen raspberries, semithawed
3 tablespoons ground flaxseeds
2–3 packets Splenda sugar substitute
1 teaspoon pure almond extract

Toss all of the ingredients into a blender and whip until smooth and creamy, about 1 minute.

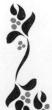

Reprinted from The Gold Coast Cure. ©*2005 Andrew Larson, M.D., Ivy Ingram Larson. Health Communications, Inc.*

3

NO PAIN . . . NO GAIN

Success consists of getting up just one more time than you fall.

Oliver Goldsmith

Slow and Steady

A pessimist sees the difficulty in every opportunity; an optimist sees the opportunity in every difficulty.

Sir Winston Churchill

"I hate to be the bearer of bad news," my doctor said, poring over my chart, "but you know about those warning signs for stroke and heart attack? Well, you have them all." In that moment, my life changed. I had avoided going to a doctor for years for just this reason. I was afraid to hear these very words. Now I had finally found the courage, and I was forced to face my worst fears.

Don't get me wrong. I knew there had to be problems. I was clearly overweight. I had been taking medication for high blood pressure for years. I was smoking and eating every bit of junk food I could lay my hands on. I was fifty-four years old when it caught up with me.

I could have received the doctor's verdict as a death sentence. Instead, I took it as a challenge. There I was, already faced with the weight and blood pressure issues, and now I had high cholesterol and borderline diabetes to deal with as well. Some changes had to be made immediately.

I started thinking about things that I needed to stop doing. Smoking was first. That stupid habit, always more of a social thing for me, was finished. The diabetes demanded that sugar had to go. That was a problem. I had always loved my sweets, and I still do. I could cut down on my fat intake, including red meat, and maybe give up white flour in the bread I loved so much. Some exercise wouldn't hurt, and perhaps a vegetable now and then would do me some good. I hated all green food.

I had tried the various popular diets. I'd done Scarsdale, Atkins and Nutri-System. They all worked, in that I lost a lot of weight on each one of them, but I gained it all back. It was clear to me that a diet wasn't what I needed. I needed to change the way I thought about my life in general, and my eating habits in particular.

I've been around long enough to know myself pretty well. I know that if I deprive myself of all of the things I love, I will quickly revert to form. I had to find a solution that would help me regain my health while still allowing me to enjoy one of my great passions, eating. It was a short drive from the doctor's office to my home. By the time I got there, I had a plan.

My plan was not low-carb. I'd done that, lost some weight and become bored. It was low-fat. That just made sense to me. It began with oatmeal topped with one half of a banana in the morning, followed by about thirty minutes of exercise. I knew that if I made the exercise routine too strenuous right off the bat I would find excuses. I needed something I would be willing to do every day. I created a little routine that involved yoga and some work with an exercise ball. Though it had some difficult features, most of the workout was about stretching. In other words, it made me feel good.

I ate a lot of chicken and turkey. I grilled some salmon once or twice a week. I filled the vegetable requirement with lots of salads that included raw vegetables. I stayed away from white bread, though I did supplement my meals with a snack of a wheat bagel now and then. I switched from sandwiches to wraps, and only wheat wraps at that. If I had tuna, I mixed it with some good olive oil instead of mayo. I tried to stay away from salt to help with my blood pressure. I developed a sensible, healthful diet that I could live with.

I don't have a scale in my house. The only way I know if I'm losing weight is by how my clothes fit, and after a couple of weeks on my new eating plan, and everyday exercise, my pants were already feeling looser around my waist. There is nothing like results to keep you on your path. If anything, my will to get healthy only intensified as the results became more apparent. I surprised myself by not only resisting temptation, but not even feeling it.

It's been about six months now. As of my last doctor's visit I had lost thirty-five pounds. I'm doing it slowly and healthily. My blood pressure is under control, my cholesterol has been cut in half and my blood sugar is close to normal. I still monitor all of these things very closely. I don't smoke, and I exercise every day.

I know that I can't go back to my old lifestyle. It's not an option for me, so there's no sense wasting time thinking about it. I feel good, and friends tell me that I look good, too. I'm not going to say that anyone can do this. In my case, it took a virtual death sentence to break me of a lifetime of bad habits. But wouldn't it be nice if you could turn it all around now, before having to hear those dreaded words from your doctor?

The key, at least for me, is moderation. Crash diets have been proven time and again to be ineffective. I needed to create a plan for myself that I could live with. I know what's good for me, and what's not. I go slow. I enjoy the way a deep stretch feels in the morning. I challenge myself and then exceed my expectations.

Ken Shane

Thin! Nine Years . . . and Counting!

I'm not overweight. I'm just nine inches too short.

Shelley Winters

There were no fat shirts available to hide the 200-plus pounds overloading my 5'1" frame. Life had happened—pregnancy, middle age, bagels and burritos. Everyone said I carried it well, but it's impossible to carry 100 excess pounds "well."

I knew the weight had to go. My health was not good, and it was time for commitment. I had tried every weight-loss program known to womankind, plus a few I invented myself. Clothing-covered relics hid in my basement—workout machines promising miracles, all unfulfilled.

I had everything to lose—100 pounds, literally! A friend was losing weight on a low-carb plan, so I headed to my local bookstore, settled into one of their comfy chairs and read everything I could find about low-carb dieting. It was time for action!

At the grocery store, I became a compulsive label reader, taking notes and memorizing the carb counts of my favorite foods. I was astounded to find that I was regularly eating in excess of 300 grams of carbohydrates per day! No wonder there was too much me! Following the plan's guidelines, I tabulated how many grams of carbohydrate I could eat in a day and made my food choices, being careful to include as many food groups as possible. The more I learned, the more food choices I included, loading up on veggies and low-carb fruits. About a month into this adventure, the comments began, "You're losing weight! Congratulations!"

I was on the way to a much thinner, healthier and happier me, but I did not become overweight overnight and could not expect to become thin quickly. It took over two years to lose 100 pounds. However, nine years into this lifestyle, the weight has not returned. My weight varies three to five pounds, one way or the other, and I wear size 6-8-10, depending on the cut of the clothing. Size 22-24 is gone forever! At a youthful fifty-four, I look like I did in my twenties, plus a few wrinkles!

This is a lifestyle change, nothing less. Lifelong weight loss requires long-term decision making. To succeed, I had to change how, what and why I ate. I had to decide what was more important—improved long-term physical and emotional health or indulging my craving for cherry pie. Instant gratification and emotional eating were contributory factors to my largesse. I finally decided I was more important than what I ate.

I approached this life change one day at a time, one meal at a time, one bite at a time, keeping in my mind's eye a thinner, healthier me. By breaking the process into small, manageable decisions, I wasn't overwhelmed by the enormity of losing 100 pounds. All I had to decide was what to do with this one bite. I planned my eating, especially in the early stages. I wrote down everything I ate, which brought awareness of the actual amount I ate, and I was shocked.

When eating out, I have a choice of two or three meals. I eat chicken frequently. I also love pork and fish. These foods, accompanied by a salad and veggies, are low-carb, delicious and I don't feel deprived. Because the protein I eat keeps me satisfied, portion control is managed well, and I rarely eat a complete meal. The three hot wings remaining on my plate will be a snack later. I never count calories, as I automatically eat less. I eat breakfast and often find it is midafternoon before I am hungry.

During my transformation I realized that the social aspects of eating are just as, or more, important than what I am eating. When my friends and I eat together, we laugh and share our lives. Mashed potatoes and gravy have taken a back seat to enjoying my friendships.

Those late-night cravings still strike, but I have predetermined foods ready to eat. Sugar-free chocolate pudding made with half-and-half, covered with whipped topping, is especially yummy at 10:00 PM. So is low-carb yogurt on low-carb cereal. Not only is this delicious, it is crunchy. You can snack—you just have to plan ahead.

When shopping, I don't stray from my route. I buy what I can eat and leave. Not only is my shopping accomplished quickly, there is very little impulse buying. On the perimeter of the store I find my dairy, veggies, fruit and meat. My only forays into the aisles are for salad dressings, sugar-free puddings, some Jell-O, or tea and coffee.

I've learned being patient with myself is vital to my success, as is having achievable expectations. It took more than forty-five years to reach my highest weight, and I had to be realistic about how long it would take to reach my goal. I also had to accept how I would look when my goal was reached. I have a medium bone structure—I will never be as small as my best friend, who is very small-boned. Sharman is the right size for her bones, and I am the right size for mine. Some things we have no control over. We keep each other on track and have made a life-long commitment to this plan and promised to encourage, as well as chastise, each other, when necessary. We exercise together frequently, walking and sharing where we are with our eating and exercise. Accountability is a good thing.

I also give myself an occasional treat. About once a month I have a toasted bagel with cream cheese, or on my son's birthday, I have a very small slice of his rhubarb pie. The next day I go right back on the plan. Special-occasion foods and small, planned indulgences keep us emotionally satisfied and moving forward.

Lifelong weight loss is a life choice. I know if I return to my former eating habits, the weight will return. I know how my body works. These principles apply to many weight-loss plans. Low-carb is the one that worked for me.

Nine years into my lifestyle change, I am healthier than ever, have more energy and my vision for the future is boundless! Accomplishing my goal has done wonders for my life view. Previously, life was shadowed by the oft-quoted phrase that inside me was a thin person screaming to get out. Well, she is out! To stay!

Linda Sago

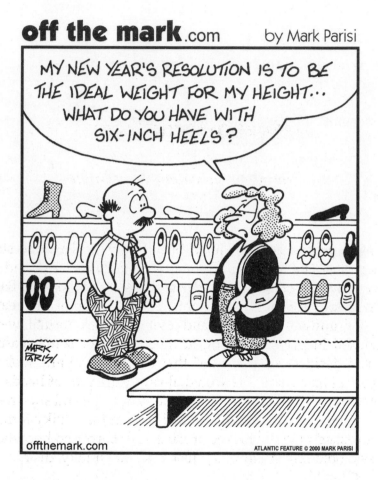

Reprinted by permission of Mark Parisi.

Peel-a-Pound Soup

Never eat more than you can lift.

Miss Piggy

The year was November 1975. Lynne and I were stationed at the American Embassy in Mexico City, and it was several weeks before the evening of the Marine Ball. This was THE most important social function of the year.

My army dress blues and Lynne's black formal were cloaked in plastic hanging in the closet. For some reason she'd decided to "try it on" that afternoon. Lynne looked great in black, and she would always turn a lot of heads at that formal event. I was very proud of my wife and she knew it. When she came out of the bedroom in that slinky formal and asked how she looked, it must have surprised her when I said (jokingly, mind you), "Just a tad bit chunky, dear."

"What?!"

Now in all honesty, I'd been sitting in the recliner half asleep while watching TV, so I wasn't alert to the possible ramifications of my remark; however, her tone of voice snapped me completely awake. "What do you mean . . . CHUNKY?"

"Uh . . . um, well, it just seems a little snug in the hips is all. Actually it looks fine, dear."

Her normally soft blue eyes glared menacingly, piercing me like an insect specimen impaled on a pin. There was no way I'd get out of this easily. It turned out I didn't have to . . . well, that's not entirely true.

The following evening I walked in the door to be met with a horrendous smell that put my olfactory senses on high alert. Lynne was in the kitchen stirring a large pot of soup. She looked up, smiling sweetly. "Hello, dear. Have a good day?" I simply nodded; relieved that apparently I was forgiven for my faux pas of the afternoon before.

"What's in the pot?" I asked, fearing her answer. As I suspected, she replied with "dinner." I stood with my mouth agape as she stirred the concoction a few more times before looking up at me and saying, "It's called Peel-a-Pound Soup. It's very filling, and since you've decided I'm a bit CHUNKY, I'm going on a diet. Julie gave me the recipe," she said as she handed me a slip of paper. I stood there and read the neat printing of Lynne's best friend.

A large can of V-8 juice, a large can of tomatoes, an entire stalk of celery, six onions, one head of cabbage, one grated carrot, and just a pinch of salt, pepper and garlic powder to taste. Boil it all up and eat as much as you want.

"But Julie must weigh 165 pounds, Lynne," I protested. "She hasn't lost an ounce since we've known her."

Lynne nodded, "Julie and I are starting this diet today."

I thought for a moment, then gathered my courage. "No dear," I replied magnanimously, "WE'RE going on this diet today. After all, if I hadn't made that stupid remark . . ." I let the sentence trail off in an attempt to gain some sympathy that I knew beforehand would not be forthcoming. I was right. She set the ladle down and gave me a big hug.

"That's so SWEET of you, darling, but YOU don't have

to, you know. YOU don't NEED this diet. You're not . . . CHUNKY!"

Women!

Now I'm a "meat and potatoes" kinda guy, and as I took my first taste of this soup, I wished I was back to eating C rations in the field. The stuff was awful, but if this was what she wanted, so be it. It was the least I could do to make up for criticizing her looks. Since digestion of this soup is supposed to consume more calories than it contains, it couldn't take long until she lost the maybe five pounds it would take to make her feel comfy again. How long could this last? A couple of days at the most? Knowing her the way I did, I figured she'd get tired of this very soon, especially since it was a morning, noon and nighttime drill. In the meantime I'd grab a few rolls for breakfast at work, then eat a hearty lunch and late-afternoon snack at the restaurant next door to the embassy and wouldn't have to consume much of this god-awful concoction at home. Just enough to let her know she had my support. Anyway, that was The Plan.

The thing is, I felt guilty doing it, knowing my wife was at home eating that horrible soup while I pigged out on sweet rolls for breakfast and enchiladas for lunch. The little devil on my left shoulder whispered in my ear that it was her decision. I didn't need to lose weight, did I? Of course not! But the little angel on my right shoulder whispered that this entire situation was my fault. After all, I just needed to eat one meal of the stuff while Lynne had to choke down three of them.

Seven days and a loss of eight pounds later the diet was over. I knew it the day Lynne greeted me at our door dressed in her black formal and high heels, with the diamond pendant that I'd given her on our anniversary two years ago adorning her neck. "See?" she said, beaming, "it worked." She turned around slowly and I couldn't help but think how lucky I was to be married to such a beautiful woman.

That night we celebrated with dinner at a fancy restaurant and an evening of dancing. Both of us turned down the soup course.

Gary Luerding

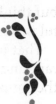

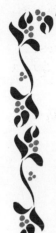

Anytime Soup

MAKES 8 SERVINGS
EACH SERVING: 5 GRAMS PROTEIN, 10 GRAMS CARBOHYDRATE

1 pound chicken parts or soup bones
½ head shredded green cabbage
1 minced garlic clove
2 chopped celery stalks
2 pounds diced fresh tomatoes
3 chopped carrots
2 tablespoons chopped fresh parsley
½ teaspoon dried thyme (optional)
½ teaspoon dried basil (optional)
freshly ground black pepper to taste
4 cups low-sodium chicken stock, or 4 cups water
2 tablespoons fresh lemon juice, or 2 tablespoons cider
    vinegar

In a large heavy-bottomed soup pot, bring all
the ingredients except lemon juice or vinegar to a
boil. Lower heat and simmer 1 hour. Remove
chicken parts or soup bones. Shred chicken and
return to pot. Add lemon juice or vinegar. Taste,
and adjust seasonings.

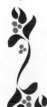

Reprinted from The Schwarzbein Principle Cookbook. ©*1999*
Diana Schwarzbein, M.D., Nancy Deville and Evelyn Jacob.
Health Communications, Inc.

Running from a Diabetic Coma to the Marine Corps Marathon

Many people limit themselves to what they think they can do. You can go as far as your mind lets you. What you believe, you can achieve.

Mary Kay Ash

I had been overweight—obese even—but I had no idea I had diabetes until I nearly died. Just after Memorial Day 2001, I started feeling nauseated. I called in sick that Wednesday and Thursday. When I didn't show up for work or call in on Friday, my manager called my father.

My dad drove from Greencastle, Pennsylvania, to Washington, DC, where he found me unconscious on the floor of my apartment. Firefighters rushed me to the emergency department at Georgetown University Hospital where I was admitted in a diabetic coma. When I regained consciousness a week later, doctors told me I had diabetes and would have to take insulin twice daily for the rest of my life.

I was in bad shape then—my muscles had so atrophied

I could barely stand and couldn't walk. They sent me by ambulance to Mount Vernon Rehabilitation Center in Alexandria, Virginia. That first day of physical therapy was agony. Pain shot up my legs. It would go on for another two weeks. When it was done, I had spent over a month in hospitals.

The night before I left rehab, one of the nurses came to see me. He was a small, wiry Southern man and an extremely professional nurse. "Remember, there's nothing you can't do," he said. I always figured he meant that literally, although I was still very sick and spent the next two months in diabetes education, examinations and more physical therapy. On my first attempt to walk the block around my apartment, I couldn't even make it to the corner. I walked a little farther every morning until I could make it to the Metrobus stop on Wisconsin Avenue and back to my apartment.

After Labor Day, I went back to work nearly thirty pounds lighter and began my life as a middle-aged poster boy. I followed through with every doctor's appointment or blood test and walked daily—forty-five minutes on weekday mornings and an hour or longer on weekends. I finished physical therapy and wanted to build upon my gains. I joined a gym and worked out three nights a week. The first night I could barely bench-press the barbell without any weight plates. I scoured local stores for books about diabetes. I began carefully planning meals and snacks. Despite everyone's doubts, I began to think I might get off of insulin. Seven times a day, I stuck my finger and tested my blood sugar. It began to come down, as did my weight. Soon I was thirty, then forty pounds lighter. After the New Year, the endocrinologist was skeptical but agreed to let me try diet control. Just eight months after the coma, I was off of insulin and all diabetes medications.

Seeking a new challenge, I entered the registration lottery for the Marine Corps Marathon. When I got the e-mail confirming my race entry, I knew that if I was going to do this I needed to join a training group. I chose the National AIDS Marathon Training Program, which raised funds for a local clinic. Although almost pathologically shy, I thought I might make a good fund-raiser, and I reached out to colleagues, family and friends with fund-raising appeals.

Recovering from a diabetic coma was the hardest thing I'd ever done. Training for the marathon was a close second. We began the first weekend in May—six months before the marathon. We met in Georgetown early Sunday mornings and ran the C&O Canal towpath. They put us into pace groups based on our expected marathon finish times. I continued training and raised almost double the fund-raising minimum.

Marathon day in late October was a blast. We drew energy from cheering crowds lined along the route. Because it started out cooler than normal, I forgot to drink water, and near the twenty-mile mark along the Mall, my calf muscles began cramping. Pain gripped me with each stride, but after all I had been through, I couldn't give up. Walking most of the rest of the way, a woman in my pace group helped me get to the Fourteenth Street Bridge before it re-opened to traffic. I did it! I finished! I was now a marathoner, who just happened to have type 2 diabetes. I crossed the finish line with a whole new outlook on life, thankful for my rapid recovery and ready to live!

Guy Burdick

What's the Point?

I can resist everything, except temptation.

Oscar Wilde

The women in my family have been living by a number system for the past several weeks, so the other day I decided to get in on the program, too. This program now assigns every edible item on the face of the earth a corresponding point value, and according to your present weight, you get a preset number of points (or food) that you can eat. Therefore, if you're lucky, that means you can have three meals a day . . . as long as you don't mind gum for one of them.

The points add up quickly. For example, a slice of bread is 2 points, an enchilada is 9 points, and a meal at McDonalds is 1,229,789—or better yet, your last meal on earth.

The night before my diet was set to start, I checked out the chart to see how many points I could eat each day. Based on my weight, I'm allowed twenty-five. Seeing as that wouldn't work for me, I decided that because I'm a man, and therefore I have the role of hunter-gatherer in the family, I should have extra points. So I gave myself thirty points a day. In other words, I added up the equivalent of twenty-five points and realized that if I stuck to that meager plan, I wouldn't be able to operate heavy machinery. But don't think that extra seven points buys me a trip down the buffet line. There are only degrees of starvation.

Actually, I did think that the first day went fairly smooth—mostly, I guess, because the night before the diet, I binged as a farewell to my old eating habits and woke up the next day barely able to walk. Still, by evening, I was starving. So my wife asked me how many points I had left for dinner. I rolled my eyes.

"I have enough to enjoy a tablespoon of dirt," I answered, "as long as there aren't any bugs (five points) in it . . . or mulch (nine points)."

The diet has gone downhill from there. To be successful, you really have to learn how to space your points out evenly throughout the day. That way, by dinnertime, you still have enough so you don't get a hunger headache, or your stomach doesn't rumble and frighten small children.

There's a discipline to the program, which, incidentally, my wife is really good at following. Just yesterday morning she was bragging about it.

"I banked three points yesterday," she announced.

I looked up from licking the bottom of my cereal bowl. "What does that mean?"

"I didn't use three points," she exclaimed.

I wanted to cry. "I'll give you ten dollars for them."

"You can't buy MY points," she answered.

"Why not?" I argued, "You're not using them."

"Yes I am," she retorted. "I can apply them to my points today. I'm going to have a latte with my lunch."

"Yum," I said. "I'll give you five dollars just to smell your breath."

I think I might have to up my daily points—like maybe by 1,229,789.

Ken Swarner

The Road to Self-Worth

One must eat to live, and not live to eat.

Molière

I am the behind-the-scenes writer of a column for a national health and fitness magazine that focuses on success stories about weight loss. For years I have written about other people and their journey to a healthy body, mind and spirit. But I've never written my own success story. Sure, I've lost ninety-five pounds and have lowered my body fat from I don't even know how high to healthy, and dropped dress sizes from 24 to 10, but I always felt like that wasn't really me.

I wasn't always overweight. Until age five, I was a healthy, active kid. It wasn't until my parents started having problems that resulted in a divorce that I turned to food. I struggled with my weight all through my school years and into college, where I reached 260 pounds during my senior year. Today, more than a decade later, people don't believe that I ever weighed that much. Even I have to pull out the before pictures to remember, and they are shocking because back then I never looked in mirrors. I never looked other people in the eye for fear of what they would say about me. I was shy. I was ashamed. I was depressed. I was scared.

Like most of the people I interview for stories, I tried all the fad diets. My parents put me on them when I was a kid, and I forced myself on them as a teen and young adult. What I didn't realize was that the worst thing I could do was to use food as a form of punishment. It would never work. And it didn't.

One dark night before graduation, I looked at my body and imagined myself at eighty-five years old. If I continued walking the path I was on, who would I be? What would I look like? I saw overweight. I saw health problems. I saw loneliness and unresolved emotional pain. I didn't like what I saw. I remembered what an old college professor said to me when I asked her for advice. She merely shrugged and said, "You just have to choose."

I got mad at her. What kind of advice is that? Choose what? How can I choose? Then it clicked. It was a mental trick. All I had to do was choose the picture of who I wanted to be at eighty-five. All I had to do was choose to allow the real me to come out of her cocoon by making small, little choices in support of my decision every single day. I would deny myself nothing. I would choose to become the best me possible. I would choose health over habit. I would choose action over inertia. I would choose love over self-loathing.

I read the health books. I got educated. I learned balance. I went for walks. I chose to eat healthy and to not completely deny myself the things I loved, but I chose to eat them less often. And I chose to see it not as a short-term, quick fix that would make me skinny tomorrow. I chose to see it as a lifelong journey to health. With the help of long walks and yoga, I learned how to listen to what my body wanted instead of the old tapes that made me crave sugar and junk food to numb out with.

It took a decade to lose that weight. I continue to lose a few pounds every year. I continue to listen to my body's needs. I know it needs sleep and downtime and play and inspiring work. I know that it needs good friends and healthy foods to fuel the things it wants to do. I know it needs movement and plenty of time outside.

Most of all I know that it needs gentle kindness and love from me. Not brutality. Losing weight over such a long time was like the proverbial herding of cats. Very gently, calmly and lovingly I would bring myself back to my goal of a healthy life each time I turned down a side road. I continue to gently shepherd my mind, body and spirit down my path to health. It's a road that I'll walk my entire life with love and gratitude, because I am and have always been worthy.

Jacquelyn B. Fletcher

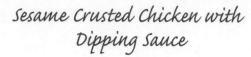

Sesame Crusted Chicken with Dipping Sauce

MAKES 4 SERVINGS
EACH SERVING: 1.5 GRAMS SATURATED FAT

extra virgin olive oil cooking spray
1 piece whole grain bread, broken into bite-sized pieces
1 tablespoon extra virgin olive oil plus 1 teaspoon
3 tablespoons sesame seeds
1 tablespoon wheat germ
⅛ teaspoon salt, plus more to taste
⅛ teaspoon cayenne pepper
½ teaspoon paprika, divided
1 pound boneless, skinless chicken breasts (pound thin)
¼ cup prepared hummus
2 tablespoons canola oil mayonnaise
1 teaspoon Tabasco (or other hot sauce)
1 tablespoon lemon juice

Preheat oven to 400° and coat a baking dish with cooking spray. In a food processor or blender, add the whole grain bread, 1 tablespoon of the olive oil, sesame seeds, wheat germ, ⅛ teaspoon salt, cayenne pepper, and a ¼ teaspoon of paprika; pulse to make fine crumbs, about 1 minute. Transfer crumbs to a large Ziplock plastic bag.

In a medium-sized bowl, toss chicken in teaspoon of olive oil and season with salt to taste. Add chicken, one piece at a time, to the bag and coat both sides with the crumbs. Transfer chicken to the baking dish. Bake for 15–18 minutes, or until cooked through.

Whisk together the hummus, mayonnaise, Tabasco, lemon juice and remaining ¼ teaspoon of paprika. Remove chicken from oven and transfer to a platter. Serve immediately with dipping sauce on the side.

Reprinted from Fitter, Firmer, Faster. ©2006 *Andrew Larson, M.D., Ivy Ingram Larson. Health Communications, Inc.*

READER/CUSTOMER CARE SURVEY

We care about your opinions! Please take a moment to fill out our online Reader Survey at **http://survey.hcibooks.com**.
As a **"THANK YOU"** you will receive a **VALUABLE INSTANT COUPON** towards future book purchases as well as a **SPECIAL GIFT** available only online! Or, you may mail this card back to us and we will send you a copy of our exciting catalog with your valuable coupon inside.

First Name _____ MI. _____ Last Name _____

Address _____

State _____ Zip _____ City _____ Email _____

1. Gender
❑ Female ❑ Male

2. Age
❑ 8 or younger
❑ 9-12   ❑ 13-16
❑ 17-20   ❑ 21-30
❑ 31+

3. Did you receive this book as a gift?
❑ Yes   ❑ No

4. Annual Household Income
❑ under $25,000
❑ $25,000 - $34,999
❑ $35,000 - $49,999
❑ $50,000 - $74,999
❑ over $75,000

5. What are the ages of the children living in your house?
❑ 0 - 14   ❑ 15+

6. Marital Status
❑ Single   ❑ Married
❑ Divorced ❑ Widowed

7. How did you find out about the book?
(please choose one)
❑ Recommendation
❑ Store Display
❑ Online
❑ Catalog/Mailing
❑ Interview/Review

8. Where do you usually buy books?
(please choose one)
❑ Bookstore
❑ Online
❑ Book Club/Mail Order
❑ Price Club (Sam's Club, Costco's, etc.)
❑ Retail Store (Target, Wal-Mart, etc.)

9. What subject do you enjoy reading about the most?
(please choose one)
❑ Parenting/Family
❑ Relationships
❑ Recovery/Addictions
❑ Health/Nutrition
❑ Christianity
❑ Spirituality/Inspiration
❑ Business Self-help
❑ Women's Issues
❑ Sports

10. What attracts you most to a book?
(please choose one)
❑ Title
❑ Cover Design
❑ Author
❑ Content

TAPE IN MIDDLE; DO NOT STAPLE

NO POSTAGE
NECESSARY
IF MAILED
IN THE
UNITED STATES

BUSINESS REPLY MAIL

FIRST-CLASS MAIL PERMIT NO 45 DEERFIELD BEACH, FL

POSTAGE WILL BE PAID BY ADDRESSEE

Chicken Soup for the Dieter's Soul
3201 SW 15th Street
Deerfield Beach, FL 33442-9875

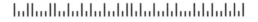

FOLD HERE

Comments

Do you have your own Chicken Soup story
that you would like to send us?
Please submit at: **www.chickensoup.com**

Stop Dieting, Start Living

*A*rgue *for your limitations and sure enough they're yours.*

Richard Bach

I was overweight by the time I was five—chubby, with red hair and freckles. It wasn't anybody's fault, just a series of circumstances that set me on a roller coaster.

As a child, I learned not to waste food. There were "starving children in Africa," so I dutifully cleaned my plate. I had a skinny, athletic brother who ate anything that wasn't nailed down, and I rushed to get my share first. From my grandmothers, who were both wonderful cooks, I learned that food was love.

At nine, my parents divorced, and I discovered security and comfort in eating. As a teenager, I dealt with boredom by baking—and eating—chocolate chip cookies and hanging out at fast-food joints with my friends. Over time, my faithful friendship with food became a love/hate relationship. I was caught in a free fall of eating to meet my emotional needs.

I first became aware that I was fat at six, when my dad

teased me about swallowing a watermelon seed. By eleven, embarrassing shopping trips to find clothes confirmed that I needed to lose weight. My mother was slender and I never saw her eat a baked potato like the rest of us. I always knew that eventually, I wouldn't get to have them anymore either. For the next twenty years, I rode that roller coaster of overeating and dieting.

It was never-ending: guilt when I ate what I wanted, deprivation when I ate what I was allowed to. I tried to be "good," but it didn't last. I used exercise to earn extra calories and pay penance when I was "bad." As a result, whenever I quit dieting, I quit exercising too. I was ashamed of my body, my eating and my cheating. Dieting caused steeper climbs and deeper drops. I felt like I was careening out of control.

Despite my lack of success with dieting, I did well in college and medical school. During my residency, I delivered tiny babies in the middle of the night, resuscitated dying people in the emergency room and assisted in long operations with cranky attending surgeons. The only saving grace was the free food in the cafeteria. I deserved it.

At any time of the day or night, I found company in the doctors' lounge and comfort in the special-of-the-day. It didn't take me long to discover the double-dipped malted milk balls in the bulk bin. A wax paper sackful slipped into my white coat pocket would last me all night. Each little chocolate sphere was a consolation prize that gave me the confidence, energy, reward and pleasure I desperately needed. I gained a lot that first year—a whole new resilience and spirit—and at least ten pounds in malted milk balls.

When it was over, I started another round of self-denial. The clackety-clack up the hill felt good. "I'm finally back in control," my little voice said. I weighed myself and calculated how long it would take to reach my goal. I cleaned out my refrigerator, kitchen cabinets and desk drawer. I threw away (or finished off) all the "bad" stuff, started eating celery sticks for snacks and drank my eight glasses of water every day. I read labels so I'd know what I could eat and stopped going out to dinner. I bought new walking shoes and got up early every morning. "You can do it this time!" my little voice said.

The weight started to come off. I lost four pounds that first week. Never mind that part of it was water or even muscle. I already felt thinner—and a little smug. I was near the top of the hill, watching everyone below scarfing down junk food.

Then one day I weighed in and I hadn't lost as much as I thought. I vowed to try harder, and I did, for awhile. My little voice whispered, "This isn't worth it." I saw someone eating ice cream and I heard, "It's not fair." I woke up early for my walk, but it said, "This is too hard." I went back to sleep.

Time stood still as I crested the hill. I bought a bag of Hershey's Kisses and had it open before I left the parking lot. I was picking up speed. The little voice said, "You can walk extra tomorrow. Have another one." I ate one more, then another, and before I knew it, half the bag was gone. My little voice repeated the familiar phrase, "You already blew it. You might as well eat the rest so you won't be tempted when you go back on your diet tomorrow." Besides, how was I going to explain half a bag of candy?

The exhilaration didn't last long. By that evening, my little voice was taunting me, "You're a loser!" I vowed to be good, but I knew I was just one piece of chocolate away from losing control again. It seemed I'd bought a lifetime ticket.

What was wrong with me? How could I practice medicine and raise a family, but fail at dieting? I knew most of my patients weren't having much long-term success either. Maybe it wasn't me.

My husband and children never dieted and never struggled with their weight. In fact, they ate whatever they wanted, but they rarely ate more than they needed.

Did they just have better metabolisms than I did? That was probably part of it. I knew mine was a mess after years of overeating and dieting. Did they have more willpower? No. I doubted they could stay on a diet for very long either. But there was something fundamentally different about the way they thought about food. In fact, they didn't really think about food at all—unless they were hungry.

Could the answer really be that obvious? Could I use hunger again to guide my eating, instinctively? My only other choice was to strap myself in for another ride. My little voice screamed, "I want off!"

So I jumped. No more rules, no more deprivation, no more sneak eating.

It wasn't easy at first. Years of ignoring hunger and fullness while I ate to meet my emotional needs or follow the latest diet rules made it hard to trust my body and my instincts. But I slowly discovered that when I took the time to tell the difference between body hunger and head hunger, I was able to better meet both my physical and emotional needs.

I gave my little voice a new mantra: "Eat when you're hungry, stop when you're satisfied." Even now, it reminds me, "When you eat food your body didn't ask for, it will store it," and, "There will always be enough food, so there's no reason to eat it all now."

Instead of drastic ups and downs, I try to balance eating for health with eating for enjoyment. I use balance, variety and moderation to guide my eating instead of harsh, complicated rules. Now I can enjoy cooking, dining out and eating with friends. I feel my best when I'm nourishing my body and my soul.

I also love to hike and do yoga several times a week, not to control my weight but for the stamina, strength, flexibility and calm they give me. I've found peace, health and wholeness. I've also discovered a purpose for my life and a passion for helping others get off their roller coaster, too.

I knew my long ride was finally over when my husband gave me a sack of double-dipped malted milk balls and it took me a week to eat them. Even though I still love chocolate, it's not my best friend anymore.

Michelle May, M.D.

One Newspaper at a Time

*Imprisoned in every fat man a thin one is wildly
signaling to be let out.*

Cyril Connolly

One of the unfortunate side effects of being very overweight is constant back pain. Sitting, standing, lying
down, carrying, lifting . . . no matter what the activity, my
back is always in some state of pain.

Recently, I decided to do something about this. Not
only did I want to relieve the back pain that carrying
around an extra 150 pounds creates, I also wanted to head
off all the other medical problems I knew were in my
future. My biggest concern was exercise. How could I possibly move this bulk of mine around when I was already
in pain? Stretching, jogging, lifting weights and all the
other activities that I knew would help get the weight off
just seemed impossible to do with my back always feeling
like it was twisted in a knot.

So I started out slowly. I got a paper route, which to be
honest was not a weight-loss strategy at first. However,
after I signed up, I found out that I had to porch all of the

papers. This meant that I had to get out of my car (YIKES!) and physically walk the paper up the driveway and place it on the porch. This may not sound tough to many people, but to a 300-pound woman the thought of getting in and out of a car and walking up and down forty-seven driveways didn't sound fun. And I just knew this would aggravate my back to the point that I wouldn't be able to move at all.

Day one came and I got in and out of my car and I huffed and puffed up forty-seven driveways at two in the morning—and I sweat like I hadn't in years. I hauled myself home, got in bed and went back to sleep. When I woke up several hours later, I sat up and realized that not only was my back not throbbing in pain, as I had thought it would, but it actually felt a little bit looser.

Each week I noticed my back pain getting progressively less. Well, I figured that if just walking a little every day could help, maybe adding in a little extra exercise would help even more. I took it easy, a little at a time, doing simple exercises and other activities like playing with my children instead of popping in yet another movie for them to watch. And here came another side effect. I started to lose a little weight. As the weight came off, the back pain lessened.

I had always thought that I couldn't exercise because I was too large. The pain in my body, along with the sheer bulk of me, was simply too much to put through any kind of a workout routine. If I did manage to exercise, I just knew I would be in agonizing pain the next day. But just the opposite happened. This amazing human body began to function better the more I exercised. Logic had always told me that if I lost weight, my back wouldn't hurt so much. After all, 300 pounds is a lot of weight for one back to carry. But the task of losing that weight just seemed too much to conquer.

So now I'm taking baby steps. I have created a mental

picture of me, newspaper carrier that I am, with 150 news-papers, each weighing a pound, strapped to my back. Every time I lose a pound, it's like I'm throwing away one of those newspapers. Each time I toss a paper, my health is that much better, my back pain is that much less and I'm one step closer to the healthier, happier person I want to be.

I try not to look at the whole picture—losing 150 pounds. I don't want to know how much I need to lose or how much further I want to go. If I focus on the fact that I have only delivered ten papers out of a 150-paper route, I'm going to want to just crawl in bed and never see the light of day again. So I don't focus on that. I take it slow. I allow myself to be proud of every moment I can sit without leaning over to crack my aching back, proud of every ounce I've lost and every ounce of mobility I've gained. And I just take each day as it comes, one newspaper at a time.

Michelle McLean

Joint Effort

*Have you strength enough to take this first step?
Courage enough to accomplish this small act?*

Phillipe Vernier

In the shelter of an ATM kiosk, eight soggy strangers and I waited for the rain to stop. We were in Nashville with thousands of others for the Country Music Marathon, now on rain delay. We were grouped by speed, and I was in the back with the walkers. Lightning flashed. When the danger passed, we'd be the last to know. The rest of the Joints in Motion team waited somewhere up the street. In training, we'd faced lousy weather together, but now we were apart and facing a full marathon of 26.2 miles. I hadn't planned on starting it with my windbreaker clinging to me and sore feet squishing inside my shoes.

Before I started Joints in Motion training, I had lost twenty-five pounds. It wasn't the first time. This time, though, success was critical. My doctor had me on medications for high blood pressure and cholesterol. Reducing sodium and walking for thirty minutes at work hadn't helped. Weight loss did. My doctor took me off both medications. I wanted to keep it that way. How? I decided that fitness was the key.

Joints in Motion was perfect for my needs. I wanted to finish a marathon, a huge goal and one that would burn a lot of calories. The program provides weekly training with a coach and workshops on proper nutrition, shoes, clothing and exercise. We even had access to a sports doctor if injured. Best of all, I had a team to keep me motivated. In exchange for meeting a fund-raising goal for the Arthritis Foundation, we'd get free registration and transportation to the marathon, hotel, a prerace pasta dinner, breakfast before and a team party after the event.

How better to get in shape, make friends, travel to fun places and help others at the same time? Our Nashville team ranged from college students to forty-somethings like me. Most paired up with runners who trained at similar speeds. However, I was the sole walker. I walked a fifteen-minute mile, twice the speed I'd walked with my coworkers.

Each week, the mileage grew. Cold rain fell during one run, soaking me through my poncho to the skin. Then came winter, and one memorable run at the only park where the trails weren't covered in ice. At ten below zero, the wind sliced through us. Everyone else finished. They thawed out inside the warm cars, drinking coffee. Coach Dave came out to check on me. "I don't think I can do anymore," I said. He went the last two miles with me, a bagel in one hand and cocoa in the other.

The miles increased into early spring, until the trial run for the marathon: the twenty-one miler. We followed a course along the Mississippi River through little towns. By now, the muscles in my legs and hips were well defined. I found the balance of proteins and carbohydrates that would give me enough energy for distance walking. I looked better in my clothes, thanks to having more muscle and less fat. I had the proper equipment and training to achieve the marathon. Would it be enough?

At the pasta dinner before the race, spirits were high. We sang funny songs to honor our coaches and the volunteers. The next day, however, brought unpleasant surprises. First, the rain. Then, a forty-five-minute wait for shuttles to the race start. We'd barely make it on time. But the starting time came and went. The crowd waited for the weather alert to pass, with contenders for the Athens Olympics in front, and us walkers in back. Half an hour later, we ventured onto the road. The throng of people surged forward. The marathon had begun. I jogged to the five-mile mark and then I faded back to my comfortable pace. I didn't want to burn out early.

I saw my friends occasionally. At eighteen miles, a woman had her knee wrapped at a first aid station. After that, I was on my own. The crowd thinned. Pain and fatigue set in. The long, wet wait that morning and jogging had worn me down. I plodded on, unable to keep up my pace. As mile twenty-one neared, I struggled.

The rainy morning turned into a steamy afternoon—over eighty degrees, warm for April in Tennessee. Some people succumbed to exhaustion and were transported to the finish for medical care. At mile twenty-three, sweat dried into a salty crust on my body. I drank some warm sports drink. My stomach was queasy. I nibbled a few pretzels as I hobbled along. A car slowed down alongside me. The volunteer thought I was in trouble. "Are you alright?"

"Yeah."

"You want a ride?"

I shook my head, unwilling to use my energy to speak. I wouldn't quit now. My mind was foggy; my legs jerked like a wooden puppet's, but I kept on. Some remaining walkers quickened their pace in the last mile, but I just willed myself to keep moving. Over the slapping of feet on pavement, I heard an announcer. I staggered toward the sound. I finished in six hours, fifty-one minutes.

I have finished two half-marathons and numerous shorter walks since then. Most are for charity. Some I do with the friends I made on the Nashville team. I've mentored another Joints in Motion team, training with them and helping raise funds. Now I'm the one giving out Powerade and encouragement at the twenty-one milers. I may even do another full marathon.

To keep my cholesterol and blood pressure at healthy levels, I need to keep excess weight off. Healthy eating and walking have helped me do that. The body is like the old car we bought that had spent the past five years sitting in a driveway. The belts, brake shoes, water pump and more had to be replaced, simply because the car had been idle. Likewise, the body breaks down if fluids are pooling instead of pumping, levers are stiff from disuse and whole systems are allowed to rust. If I am always training for another event, I am keeping in my active habits. At the same time, I am making friends and helping people who I will never meet. It's a win/win for everyone.

Debra Weaver

Dieter's Block

Success is going from failure to failure without loss of enthusiasm.

Winston Churchill

I want to achieve a healthy weight, really I do. But in recent years, I have been losing the battle of the bulge. Like millions of other Americans, I have watched the numbers creep up. It's not just my weight, but the size of my clothes. And don't even get me started on things like cholesterol and blood pressure. Aren't things that go up supposed to come down? Fortunately, I have discovered the cause of my weight gain: I have dieter's block.

Dieter's block can be triggered by a variety of things, circumstances that the ordinary mortal, such as me, simply cannot control. Perhaps the day is too cold or too warm. Or maybe the weather is perfect and practically begs the eating of a double-fudge sundae. It could be the need for caffeine that drives me to order a large café mocha, extra-sweet, extra-hot. Every day. Twice.

Sometimes it is that special occasion that seems to pop up right after I have made yet another vow to cut back, cut down, cut it out! It could be a favorite sister's birthday, a friend's promotion or a child who needs consoling after a big game. Nothing says comfort like a grilled cheese sandwich and tomato soup, peach pie with ice cream, or homemade chicken and dumplings. Yum.

Of course, there is always exercise. My dieter's block interferes with my exercising all the time. Experts always say you should not work out within an hour before eating or two hours after eating. Do these experts have no life? The way my schedule has been lately, I have exactly seven and a half minutes a day that is safe for me to exercise. With a two-hour commute and an hour for lunch added to an eight-hour day, it always seems that other things lay claim to those precious minutes, and I tell myself, "I'll start tomorrow."

Dieting has become a way of life for many people. Who can blame them? There is a diet designed to fit almost any need: low-carb, low-fat, low-calorie, the list goes on. If you are not fond of veggies, go with the high-protein, low-carb diet. If you can't stand the thought of eating meat, do the vegan thing. Skip meals, add meals. There is truly something for everyone. The only drawback is . . . you actually have to do the diet. There's where my dieter's block gets in the way again.

I am a great one for talking about a diet, or planning a diet, but actually dieting? That will take some doing. Today's not a good day, you know, we had a company-wide meeting with refreshments. I had to participate, it's part of my job. I can't start on Friday; everyone knows the weekend is a terrible time to start a diet. Maybe Monday. But Mondays are so harsh. What an awful day to start a diet. Tuesday? Doesn't someone have a birthday on Tuesday? Didn't I promise to bring cookies?

Terry A. Lilley

Jiggles

A waist is a terrible thing to mind.

Tom Wilson

Only Jell-O is supposed to jiggle.

But any overweight person knows that a whole lot of shaking goes on before a bountiful body becomes a lean, dream, fit machine. Instead of benefiting from the physics of exercise equipment and the knowledge of personal trainers, many dieters never set foot inside a gym or health club.

If life were fair, consistently exercising smart food choices would be the only activity needed to rid the body of the bulges that wiggle and jiggle.

But life isn't fair, as my whining children often hear. I had to eat those words myself when my naturally slender friend, Barb, unknowingly fed them to me.

Until that day, I'd assumed her model figure came naturally. It had, the self-proclaimed junk food lover said while eating a dinner salad. But when she hit middle age, gravity began pulling at her butt, boobs and midsection as relentlessly as it tugged at the rest of us. And her junk food diet started adding on unwanted pounds.

Instead of joining the chorus of whiners bemoaning the injustice of gravity and slowing metabolisms, she moved to counter nature's effects.

Literally.

She began rising before the sun, getting in forty-five minutes of aerobics and weight training in the quiet comfort of home while the alarm clock let her family sleep until 5:00 AM.

Completing this morning ritual is now as automatic as keeping her weekly manicure appointments. Fair or not, she said, it's what she has to do to maintain the look she wants.

Aha! I thought, swallowing more than the last of my dessert.

With enlightened resignation, I pledged to get physical once again. This time, though, the pledge was sealed with a commitment to hang tough over the long haul. Long enough to see whether exercise coupled with my diet would work for me, too.

Early morning walks along neighborhood streets more familiar to the wheels of my car than to the soles of my feet were the start. Then, apprehension following a close encounter with deer made me retreat to my home. I did aerobic video workouts and calisthenics using hand weights or the natural heft of my body parts.

The euphoria of my new commitment propelled me day to day from tape to tape for a while; so did disdain for the jiggles and the girdles, now called body shapers, marketed to keep bouncing bodies in check. Feeling tight and toned was my long-term goal.

Completing a ninety-minute aerobics tape without panting like a puppy was the short-term one. It loomed large, like an Olympian challenge far out of reach.

But it wasn't.

My fitness pledge fueled a new morning ritual. Whether a leap or a crawl moved me out of bed, the video trainer put me through my paces every weekday. Before sunrise, just like Barb.

In time, I was running out of tape long before I ran out of breath.

And the jiggles came to an end.

I still remember glowing in the gold medal moment of that realization.

It was a typical morning, except that instead of wearing the spandex leotard that helped me pretend my muscles were taut, I wore a sports bra and cotton briefs. This out-fit revealed the first signs of the change taking shape—the waistband was loose and the seat was baggy.

There were other changes, too. I was stepping higher during marches in place because a big belly no longer blocked the lift of my knees. My butt didn't bounce when I stopped moving and my flexed arms showed definition from biceps toning up.

The jiggles were gone.

Of course, none of it happened overnight. Diet and exercise progress in incremental bites must have fed my commitment subconsciously any time the lure of the pillow threatened to smother the lure of physical fitness.

A full plate of changes still feeds my commitment to the lifestyle changes I've made, including:

- Seeing boobs, not stomach, when looking down toward the floor. Feeling hip bones, not love handles, when my arms are by my side.
- Having oversized T-shirts and sweatshirts glide over my hips, not bunch at my waist. Getting more days from my pantyhose because thunder thighs aren't rubbing holes in them.
- Realizing leggings should not feel like girdles.

- Walking around naked at day's end without seeing telltale underwear marks.
- Wearing form-fitting workout gear, not loose, extra large anything, even at home alone.

No, life isn't fair, especially the dieter's life. Now I know it takes the consistency of smart food choices and regular exercise to banish the bulges that bug me. It's a combination I pledge to continue so that all that jiggles is my Jell-O.

Edwina L. Kaikai

The Exercise Bike

Those who do not find time for exercise will have to find time for illness.

Earl of Derby

I caught a glimpse of myself in a full-length mirror at the mall last Tuesday. On Wednesday, I introduced my credit card to the nice man at the fitness outlet.

Finding the perfect exercise bike took a bit of effort. It had to have a nice, big seat. And if I was going to be riding it everyday, I may as well buy one of the air resistance models. That way, as I ride, I can blow my hair at the same time. It would have to be black to match my stair stepper machine/coat rack and would definitely have to be equipped with a calorie counter. This way, I could see how many chocolate bars I had earned . . . I mean burned, each time I rode.

My investment did not arrive preassembled. It was packaged in a huge, flat box and weighed approximately 700 pounds. Getting the unit into the minivan was one thing; getting it out and into the house was an adventure. I slid it out the side door and then turned to open the gate, which anyone with half a brain would have done before unloading their cargo. The latch promptly gouged me in the side, and I got my left thumb tangled in the chain link. After much struggle, I finally made my way to the front steps. Halfway up I had to stop and rest, and I prayed that none of my neighbors were watching me. I like to make people laugh, but sledding down the front steps while screaming and sitting on top of a box wasn't exactly what I had in mind.

Once I had it inside and was able to pry through those gigantic staples, I could see why it had been packed in such a large carton. Inside I found a hundred bike parts and twice that many pieces of cardboard and Styrofoam. So the floor of my office is littered with nuts, bolts, tools, bike parts and dozens of tiny cardboard chunks. I picked up the instructions, and right then I knew I was in big trouble. There, on the paper, was a parts list a mile long and a picture of a bike with ten thousand arrows pointing here and there. Worst of all, not a word of the instructions was printed in a language I could read.

I sat with a pair of pliers in one hand and a cookie in the other, wondering how I was ever going to get the stupid thing put together so I could start burning some calories. Putting the seat on was the easy part: just put two pieces together and tighten the knob. When it came to assembling the moving parts, I had a little more trouble. I had to turn the bike upside down and hold it in place with one knee while I held the pedal on with my shoulder and tightened all the coordinating nuts and bolts. It fell over three times, leaving a mark on my wall and a bruise on my leg, and by this point, I figured I had burned at least 100 calories, so I ate another cookie.

The right pedal wasn't any easier, but I managed it without further injury. After half an hour, I stood the bike upright, feeling quite proud of myself. Then, glancing at the diagram, I realized I'd forgotten a few steps. I was supposed to put the handlebars and rods on first, then the pedals last. So once again, the bike was turned over and I was taking it apart. Note: It was at this point that I closed the door to my office. I had just spent all my money on a new bike, and the last thing I needed was to have the kids rush in and demand that I start putting quarters in the "bad words" jar.

I had been home with my new purchase for a total of two and a half hours. Within that time, I had assembled and reassembled it three times, screamed at the cat, scraped my knuckles, acquired numerous bruises and eaten nine peanut butter cookies. I was fatigued and sweaty and decided this was probably the best workout I'd ever had. I stood back and admired my handy work. Everything was put together perfectly; it looked great, and I could hardly wait to ride it. But I was too tired.

The next morning when I got up, my muscles ached and I noticed the shiner that the bike had left on my leg. But I was not discouraged. I always heard that exercise was best in the mornings before eating, so I didn't have a bite. I fixed the kids some breakfast and began my leisurely ride. I hiked my ankle-length nightgown up to my knees and climbed onto the seat. Peddling steadily, I watched the calorie counter mark my progress. The children rolled their eyes at me as they left for school, but I barely noticed. I just rode and rode, feeling very proud of myself and wondering if Richard Simmons exercised in his jammies, too.

Ann Morrow

4

INSIGHTS
AND
REVELATIONS

That which we persist in doing becomes easier—not that the nature of the task has changed, but our ability to do has increased.

Ralph Waldo Emerson

Weight in the Balance

Health is not a condition of matter, but of mind.

Mary Baker Eddy

"You're having twins, aren't you?" the woman at the checkout counter smiled and asked.

"No, just one," I replied.

"Oh," she said after a long pause, while she stared at my midsection. Then she turned abruptly and started stocking the shelves behind her.

Ms. Twins wasn't the first person to ask that question during my pregnancy, nor was she the last. I attempted to brush off these comments and others like, "You shouldn't wear such bright colors, dear." Instead, I endeavored to bask in warm expectant-mother thoughts, but deep down the remarks hurt. I had a difficult time putting aside the feelings of shame and guilt that I'd felt about my weight since childhood.

I received my first diet book in junior high. My mother bought it for me because she worried over how much I "filled out" during puberty. People constantly referred to me as a "big girl." A swim coach told me to work harder since I was solid and would drop like a stone to the bottom. One guy who tried to pick me up during vacation on a cruise-by said casually that he "liked big girls."

The adolescent diet book was the first of many diets I tried throughout the years. Other diets included outright starvation (followed by bingeing, of course), pills, high fiber/grains, low-fat, no carbs, grapefruit, excessive exercise and the ever-popular divorce diet. I eventually came across a book on how people used weight gain as a buffer against events and situations in life. Armed with that knowledge, I started looking at my own life. When did I gain weight? When did I lose weight? What worked for me? I realized that I was an emotional eater. I ate to insulate myself against family friction, school and peer pressures, job stress, and unhappy relationships. Every major change in my life brought on scale tipping as well.

A few years ago, my life settled down into a steady routine. I joined a YMCA less than a mile from my home and signed up for kickboxing classes. By being vigilant, I learned how much I could eat versus how much exercise I needed to lose weight and then maintain it. No more yo-yoing up, up and down the scale. I thought I'd finally captured the balance. I felt great. I was in control. I was confident: I told myself I'd never be a "big girl" again. Then I left my job and my life as I knew it and moved back to my home state. My wonderful balance spun out of control. The combination of starting over, trying to reconform to family pressures after being away for a decade, and a whirlwind romance filled with wining, dining and ice cream sundaes with my soon-to-be husband took its toll on my newly balanced figure.

With the support of my husband, I searched for my balance again. I was heavier than I'd ever been in my life and it was a struggle. My weight yo-yoed slightly, and then I became pregnant. I was in bliss for most of the pregnancy (when people weren't making comments), anticipating the birth of my child. I told myself that it was perfectly acceptable to be heavy while I was pregnant. I had a very important job to protect and nourish my unborn child.

I gave birth to a beautiful, healthy baby girl. A bitter-sweet time followed. The joy of being a new mom was tinged in despair. My body ached. My feet hurt all the time. I felt so old and decrepit. For months I wouldn't go anywhere without my daughter. I tried to justify my weight—I wasn't just fat, I had a new baby. Hope for a quick weight loss from breastfeeding was dashed when the pounds crept down the scale agonizingly slowly, with long plateaus (contrary to what all the pregnancy books said). The old self-loathing came back as a new mantra. I felt frumpy, lumpy and wholly unattractive. My body seemed forever changed, and I was heavier than ever before.

After my daughter stopped nursing and began to eat regular food, I felt a shift in my attitude as I focused on providing her with well-balanced meals. I realized that every bite counted for her. She couldn't afford to eat wasted calories if she was going to get what she needed to grow. Her nutritional needs reminded me about balance—not only regarding food, but also physically and emotionally.

In the past I concentrated on the balance between exercise and eating for weight loss. That wasn't enough incentive for me to stay in balance. The emotional aspect had been missing. This time around I wanted to be a good role model for my daughter. To do that I needed a gentler approach, an approach that I could live with for the rest of my life and not another quick fix. For instance, controlled portions included "nondiet" food, such as dried cranberries and toasted almonds in salads and, of course, chocolate, in small, daily doses.

Once my infant grew into a toddler, exercise became a

day-by-day thing and could only be accomplished in smaller segments, like a half-hour yoga session or kickboxing video or a short walk with her around the neighborhood.

Progress has been slow and steady. I take one day at a time and continually ask myself: What do I want? What can I live with? What will keep me going? Is this something I want my daughter to emulate? This is my balance for now. I know I don't have the perfect, end-all solution for the rest of my life. What I do have, though, is the perfect solution for me at this point in time, and I hope that I can weather future change well enough to stay the course and keep my balance. A funny thing has happened, too. I feel better, not just minus aches and pains, but I feel at peace with myself, and that truly is life in balance.

Laura Schroll

Just Listen to Mom

In the long run men hit only what they aim at.

Henry David Thoreau

Mrs. Shatzel outdid herself with this spelling assignment. She asked her students to each pick a classmate, write them a letter using all twenty words in the unit and mail it to their home.

Back in the 1960s, we sixth-graders used the phone and recesses in school to stay in touch. We didn't write letters, so this assignment was a really unique experience. I couldn't wait to receive my letter in the mail, running home each day to see what the carrier had delivered. And finally, one sunny April afternoon, it arrived. I tore open the envelope, unfolded the paper and gazed at the salutation.

It read, "Dear Lard Bucket."

I never forgot how I felt reading those words. Armed with plenty of motivation but little information, I embarked on a cycle of fast, binge and surrender, repeating the same mistakes throughout my adolescence into adulthood. The spirit was willing, but the brain wasn't quite engaged.

Last year I turned forty-five and had long since entered "surrender" mode when my friend Joe proposed a friendly wager: the first to lose 10 percent of his total weight would take the other and his wife out for dinner. What did I have to lose?

So Lard Bucket accepted the wager, halfheartedly. In return, Joe gave me a copy of a fitness profile he had received from a trainer, emphasizing that the recommendations were personalized to his condition. In reading the profile and recalling dozens of past failed attempts, I was overwhelmed by the possibilities. For this round of fast and binge, should I go low-cal, high-protein, low-carb, low-fat, gym rat, diet pills, food supplements, Hollywood Bimbo Grapefruit Diet, or try one of the million variations and combinations of all of them? Or maybe it would be better to just make the dinner reservations.

That's when "the Pattern" started taking shape. It was as if Mom was painting the big picture between the lines of detail in Joe's fitness profile. Everything fit. The profile said to eat many small meals in a day; Mom always said to eat only when you're hungry. The profile said to eat "x" thousand calories per day; Mom always said never go hungry. The profile said people are hungriest in the morning; Mom always said to eat a good breakfast. The profile said Joe should lose no more than two pounds per week; Mom always said to take the weight off slowly so you won't put it back on quickly.

Mom was right all along; it was only that her advice was too general to apply without information, and now I had that.

I went to work starting with the goal itself. Saying "I need to lose the weight of an average SUV by next summer" sets you up to fail. Saying "I will lose 1.5 to 2 pounds per week, on average, every week until I reach my desired weight" becomes a recipe for success and minimizes the likelihood of a binge on the rebound.

Since you can't get discouraged if you know what to expect, there was now no fear in weighing myself every day. Weight loss is an up-and-down process. As long as the weekly average was on target, I was fine.

It took almost a year, but I have shrunk from 243 pounds to 183, from a 44 waist to a 34, and have more energy and ambition than I ever dreamed possible. Best of all, I have the knowledge and understanding needed to keep the weight off, as I have done for almost a year. And it wasn't difficult at all. I just needed to listen to Mom.

James Hammill

Spaghetti Head

Accept the things to which fate binds you, and love the people with whom fate brings you together, but do so with all your heart.

Marcus Aurelius

The sauce sat simmering for eight hours, mingling the flavors of beef, tomatoes, garlic, onions, green peppers, bay leaf and other spices. I added mushrooms and pronounced it done.

"Good," replied my young husband, "I'm starved."

The pasta was cooked al dente, so I drained it, piled it on a plate and ladled the sauce on top. Then I carried it to him, looked at his slim features . . . and DUMPED IT ON HIS HEAD. Immediately I burst into tears.

"Okay, you're done with this diet," he calmly told me with sauce dripping from his nose. He began to wipe up the mess and carry it back to the kitchen. "Call the doctor in the morning and tell him, 'No more.'"

Why would I do such a thing? Because I was starving. Literally. I was on a zero-calorie diet after I began to maintain weight on 350 calories a day. It was the 1960s and the doctor was experimenting with me. He plied me with Dexedrine to keep me going and it worked. I bounded out of bed in the middle of the night to clean closets or scrub the bathroom with great energy and intensity. Most of the time I forgot how hungry I was. But the spaghetti sauce was an old family recipe, and its aroma permeated every inch of our small house. It triggered more than just hunger—it set up a longing to be able to eat normally and a fury at those who could without adding any pounds.

Through the ensuing years I tried every diet that came along, joining thousands of others who struggle to be thin. The rice diet, grapefruit diet, liquid diet, high-fiber diet, cabbage soup diet, even the apples-only diet accompanied by an injection of urine from pregnant sheep—whatever was popular. They all worked for awhile. I just couldn't stick to them. As soon as I returned to eating what the "normal" people around me were eating, I rapidly gained the lost weight back, plus more. Why? Those starvation diets taught my body to store food for the future since it couldn't trust me to provide regular stable nutrition.

Finally, I reached the age when being thin for looks wasn't as important as my health and mobility. I was losing both and realized I needed an eating plan, not another diet. So I gathered my knowledge of diets, which was enormous by this time, and listed what worked best for me. Never get hungry. Keep plenty of healthy snacks like veggies and nuts on hand. Eat small portions more often. Enjoy fruit and simple starches in moderation. Stay away from sugars and high-starch foods. If I just HAVE to have a piece of candy or pie or cake, some macaroni and cheese or ice cream, then I have a little bit of it, savor it without guilt and go back to my new way of eating. The addition of moderate exercise and seven to eight hours of sleep each night makes my plan more successful and I'm working on both.

Am I thin? Definitely not, and I probably never will be. But I'm healthier. My tests come back from the lab with all the "right" numbers listed, pleasing my doctor. I finally enjoy my own kind of "normal." And guess what that includes? Eating an occasional plate of family-favorite spaghetti with my husband.

Jean Stewart

Half My Size

Age is strictly a case of mind over matter. If you don't mind, it doesn't matter.

Jack Benny

Nothing gets you thinking like receiving an invitation to your twentieth high school reunion. The thought of renewing relationships with people you haven't seen in ages can stimulate a negative response when you're over-weight. I received such an invitation, and while I was tempted to attend, I knew I'd have to lose many pounds before I could face anyone. After having three children in five years and being a stay-at-home mom, I had doubled in size.

I'd become an all-day grazer, reaching for goodies nonstop, and I weighed 237 pounds. My own husband weighed less than me. I'd tried diets before and sometimes opted for healthy snacks, only to have my hunger pangs control my fat-tooth and munch down on a dozen brownies and ice cream in one sitting.

Certain family members made negative comments about my weight at every picnic or holiday gathering. My husband humored me, but I could see him shaking his head as I stuffed myself with doughnuts, dip and salty chips. I just couldn't control myself. Maybe this reunion would be a goal I could commit to since my husband was adamant that we attend.

The next morning I realized I had to make a decision; he'd taken the reservation form to mail. After the kids went to school, I cried some, ate three bagels loaded with cream cheese and then made up my mind. I'd start tomorrow. I cut out a thin model from a magazine advertisement and hung her on the refrigerator as a deterrent, right next to the actual invitation.

I love to read and had books to return to the library, so on my next trip I skipped the fiction section and browsed the diet and fitness books. I ignored the clerk when she loudly said, "Someone's going on a diet," in her singsong voice. My face warmed as the other patrons standing in line stared at me.

Next, I drove to the grocery store. I selected fruits, veggies, whole-grain breads, nuts, cereals and lots of chicken. I've seen enough diet commercials to know what you should be eating. For the kids I still bought cookies and their favorite ice cream, but not mine, to help keep the temptation down. Armed with my healthy groceries, I was ready to begin day one.

That following morning for breakfast I had a healthy grain cereal with fresh strawberries and skim milk. Afterward, I chewed a mint-flavored gum and went about my vacuuming. The chewing kept me from reaching for sugary treats and kept my mouth moving. I knew that smokers used this trick to stop smoking.

I retrieved a journal I'd recently received as a gift and started to log what I ate and my beginning weight, just as the fitness book said. I also read about the importance of exercise. Motivated, all I could do at first was stroll around the block. The daily fifteen-minute walks soon turned into thirty minutes, and I even incorporated jogging. The first couple of weeks were tough; my old self wanted to admit defeat and slide backward into the comfort foods. I'd just look at that model and the invitation and know that I'd have to face everyone in eleven months. I summoned all my willpower and fought on.

My walks increased to forty-five minutes each session with one whole block of jogging every ten minutes. The walks combined with the jogging helped to ward off my constant worrying and cleared my head. I felt calmer and slept better at night. I purchased a fitness magazine and tore out some fifteen-minute workouts to target specific body areas and used them to spice up my afternoon routine.

The first twenty pounds of former baby weight came off after two months, and I was encouraged to continue, but I had eighty pounds to go. Challenging myself, I bought a ladies' bike at a local garage sale and added a thirty-minute ride to each afternoon. Each book stressed the need to exercise six or seven days each week to lose weight and only four or five to maintain. I logged in my journal everything I ate, along with the daily walks, bike rides and spot workouts.

I became consumed, goal-oriented and somewhat proud of myself. If I felt depressed, I'd step on the scale and marvel at the readings. I'd tell myself that I didn't want to cheat and ruin everything after I'd come this far.

After three months, when the second twenty pounds came off, my husband complimented me. Lucky for me the reunion was not for eight more months, because I still had sixty pounds to go. I plugged on and joined an aerobic and kickboxing class that met three nights a week. I'd stick a piece of gum in my mouth, warm up, follow the instructor and enjoy the cooldown.

It helped erase the flab and toned my body. Every day, I scribbled a vow not to cheat. Determined, I continued to munch on veggies and fruits. Along the way, I made several new friends at the class who gave me lots of nutritional advice and weight-loss hints. We established a natural camaraderie and cheered each other on. Now, not only had I lost fifty-five pounds, I had friends, which helped me restore my own personal worth.

Invigorated, I chose new tactics and began lifting weights to sculpt my muscles on my arms and legs. I found I was regaining my waistline, so I did crunches, sit-ups and even tried belly dancing on the advice of my friends. I guess I inspired my husband; he started jogging before work each morning and dropped fifteen pounds.

Ten months passed and I finally weighed in at 137 pounds. I had lost 100 pounds and met my goal! I had revitalized my inner self all because of that fateful reunion invitation. It was a wake-up call in disguise, a very healthy one. I went from a size 18 to a size 10, half my size, and I still had one month to go. That next month I weighed in at 130 pounds. I had donated all my clothes to the spouse abuse center as I decreased in size, replacing them with less expensive ones.

"Watch out stores, here I come to shop for that perfect reunion wardrobe," I said, proudly.

The reunion was a Hawaiian luau theme, so I shopped for a flowery evening gown, a new bathing suit, and a casual pantsuit and capri set. Tears slid down my cheeks as I tried on a one-piece bathing suit in a wild turquoise and lemon color, not the usual black one with the long attached skirt.

When we flew to the reunion my husband was beaming as much as I. We held hands and I felt like it was a second honeymoon as we stepped proudly into the ballroom.

"Wow, you haven't changed a bit," said Jennifer, one of

the three girls I use to hang with in high school. I was so flattered and proud inside.

"No, she hasn't, she keeps getting better all the time," said my husband, smiling. I winked at him and silently thanked him for keeping my secret.

Suzanne Baginskie

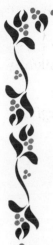

Broiled Zucchini and Feta Boats

MAKES 6 SERVINGS
EACH SERVING: 1.5 GRAMS SATURATED FAT

1 tablespoon extra virgin olive oil
1 tablespoon finely chopped garlic
3 zucchini, halved lengthwise
salt, to taste
white pepper, to taste
¼ cup low-fat feta cheese

Heat broiler. Heat olive oil in a large nonstick, ovenproof skillet (with ovenproof handle) set over medium-low heat. Add garlic and sauté for 15 seconds, or until lightly golden (be careful not to burn the garlic). Arrange zucchini halves cut side down in skillet; season with salt and white pepper to taste. Increase heat to medium and cook zucchini for 5–6 minutes, or until just carmelized (again, be careful not to let the zucchini or garlic burn).

Turn the zucchini over and season lightly with salt and white pepper; cook an additional 1–2 minutes. Arrange feta cheese on the sides of zucchini and then transfer to the broiler; broil for 2–3 minutes. Serve at once.

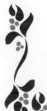

Reprinted from Fitter, Firmer, Faster. ©2006 *Andrew Larson, M.D., Ivy Ingram Larson. Health Communications, Inc.*

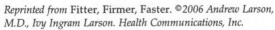

The Secret

Truth, like surgery, may hurt, but it cures.

Han Suyin

For years I searched for "The Secret" to weight loss. If I found "The Secret," then I could pass it on to my daughter and share it with the world. She and I have lost a little more than fifty pounds each. Together we've lost the equivalent of one of those little Olympic gymnasts we saw on TV. We found "The Secret."

My daughter is a wonderful example of the correct way to lose weight. She looked in the mirror one day and said to herself, "I like who I've become and what I've done with my life. I don't like the way I look; I think I'll do something about it." She found what suited her: help on the Internet. The online source for weight-loss support helped her to establish guidelines for food intake and exercise and also offered a support group for tips and advice. She stayed within the calorie, carb and fat counts outlined for her. She joined a gym and faithfully exercised three to five times a week. From April to October she steadily lost weight, going from a size 18W to a 10 Misses.

Her confidence and self-esteem zoomed through the roof.

I started last fall on what I had hoped would be my final effort to lose weight. Unfortunately, I wasn't very successful. Health problems and medications, especially the amount of insulin I was taking for diabetes, hindered my success. I finally started researching weight-loss surgery. I found a lot of information on the Internet, talked to people I knew who had had the surgery and started telling others what I was considering. People knew people who had had the surgery. I learned that weight-loss surgery is not a magic bullet but is another tool to use in a comprehensive weight-loss program. Three months ago, I decided to go for it.

I am fifty-six years old and have had problems with compulsive overeating all my adult life. My struggles with weight loss started at age six when I observed my older sister and aunt suffering as they tried to lose weight. I decided then that I never wanted to diet. When I was ten, my new stepmother let me know I was fat, and dieting became a constant in my life. Even as a teenager, when I swam and water-skied all the time, my father and stepmother kept after me to just not eat and to slim down. But nobody ever really helped me choose good foods or change my eating habits. Eventually every effort failed.

As an adult I regularly pursued whatever fad diet was popular at that time. I'd do what many do, the yo-yo thing, lose some, go off the diet, gain back more. Finally I decided to get serious help from doctors, therapists, nutritionists and God. With them in my corner, I was able to change some long-standing habits. I quit eating compulsively whenever I was feeling hurt, angry, happy or sad. I identified the roots of my feelings and learned to deal with emotions without food. The surgery has been a tool to help me complete the process. It has taken many years to get to this place. I still have 120 pounds to go to reach my goal weight. My energy level is way up; my use of medications is way down. I have gained what it takes to be successful at weight loss.

My daughter and I each, in our own way, have found "The Secret" to weight loss. "The Secret" is doing what works for you.

I would recommend her way first. Her way is the better way. My way works when diet efforts don't work—but you still have to work to reach your goal. That is why I know we will succeed and the weight will stay off: because we were, each in our own way, ready.

I have every confidence that with God's help and guidance we will both reach and maintain our goals. We are far too happy with today's results not to succeed.

Marilyn Eudaly

Seeing Double

I am an identical twin. I can look fabulous and frumpy on any given day, as people often can't tell which one of us they are talking to. Along with the benefits of having a twin sister, there is a torturous downside. The better she looks, the worse I look.

My sister and I were raised in a fairly competitive household. We were athletic in our youth and enjoyed many years of karate training and tournaments, often competing against each other. Since graduation and the births of six children between us, we have both gained and kept some unwanted pounds.

Bikini seasons, weddings and class reunions have never even come close to motivating me to lose weight as much as some good old competition with my sister. I've always been the heavier sister and I have no problem admitting it, although I'd like to point out that I'm not THAT much heavier. A goal of mine is to be lighter than my sister. I've achieved, but conceded, that goal twice, given that she was heavy with each of her daughters at the time.

My weight problem can be attributed to my love affair with white flour topped with any type of sugar: doughnuts, cakes, cookies, muffins and flavored bagels are my vices. The thought of going "carb-less" makes me shudder. Whole grains, sure, more fruits and vegetables, okay, but NO carbs, NO WAY! Getting over this "sticky" situation will surely be the key to my weight-loss success.

I have tried national diet programs, workout videos, aerobic classes, and recreational sports like softball, golf and Rollerblading to try to shed a few pounds. All of these activities died a quick death when I got sick of "counting" my food, got tangled doing the "grapevine" or got used to enjoying the cold ones after the game. My treadmill seems to be the only exercise that I enjoy. Watching the "fat grams burned" increase is more rewarding than watching the triple sevens appear on a Las Vegas slot machine.

When I finish my jog-stumble-walk on the treadmill, I realize that it wasn't all that bad, and if I can just keep the kids from joining me on the next jaunt, I might actually start seeing some results. The fact that I panted on a zero incline and at almost reverse speed proves that I am not healthy at my current weight. Nor am I happy that my sister is looking pretty good right now as a result of her minitriathlon training.

When she finishes her race, I will be there to congratulate her on her success and share in her excitement, just as she does when I have personal triumphs. Whether it is a lower number on the scale, the discovery of a great light dinner or the purchase of a new outfit from the regular-size section, I know that she'll share in my joy.

Now, if only I can figure out how to plant some nacho chips in her cupboard. They are her vice, and if she spots them, it will give me bragging rights for at least a week.

Selena Hayes

Drinking Herself Fat

*A single conversation across a table with a wise
man is worth a month's study of books.*

Chinese proverb

Determined to lose weight, my friend Julie and I started
an exercise program, which included a brisk thirty-minute
walk every morning. Julie cut her food intake to 1,500 calories a day and diligently recorded every bite she put into
her mouth in a food diary. But more than a month after
she started the strict regimen, the scale had hardly
budged.

"What's wrong with me?" she lamented one morning
after our walk. "I'm burning up more calories than I'm taking in. Why aren't the pounds melting away like they're
supposed to?" Julie opened the refrigerator and took out a
carton of orange juice. "Want some?"

I shook my head. "No, thanks. I'll just have water."

Julie poured herself a tall glass of icy-cold juice, gulped
it down and refilled the glass.

"Mind if I take a look at your food diary?" I asked.
"Maybe I can spot what's wrong."

Julie opened the drawer of her kitchen desk and took out a spiral notebook. I began reading the pages. "Do you have orange juice every day after our walk?" I asked. Julie nodded. "How come you didn't write it down?"

"I guess I never thought about writing down what I drink. I only write down what I eat."

I peered at the nutrition label printed on the side of the juice carton. "Look at this, girlfriend," I said. "Eight ounces of orange juice has 120 calories. Calories you didn't write down in that diary."

"But orange juice is so good for you," Julie said. "I usually have two glasses after I exercise. Three if I'm extra thirsty."

"That means you're taking in more calories than you burned up during the walk," I said. "And that's before you eat a bite of breakfast."

"But think of all the vitamin C."

I picked up a calorie chart that was lying on the kitchen counter and flipped to the fruit and vegetable section. "An average-size orange has only sixty calories," I read, "and fiber that the juice doesn't have. You'd be way ahead to drink water for your thirst and eat an orange for your vitamin C."

"I can't believe that never dawned on me," Julie said, a stunned look on her face.

"Let's do this," I told her. "You try to remember everything you had to drink yesterday, and I'll look up the calories."

"Two cups of coffee."

"Black?"

"No. Both cups had a big splash of flavored creamer."

"Would you say two tablespoons?"

Julie nodded.

"That's seventy calories per cup. Write down 140 in your diary. What else?"

Julie began reconstructing what she'd had to drink the

day before. There had been cereal with whole milk for breakfast, a can of cola for a midmorning pick-me-up, another when her energy began to sag late in the afternoon and bottled water with lunch.

"What about dinner?"

"Two slices of thin-crust veggie pizza."

"That's in here," I told her, studying the diary. "What did you wash it down with?"

"A wine cooler. Strawberry."

"Did you have anything to drink after dinner?"

"Well . . . I'm pretty sure I had a mug of hot chocolate while I watched TV. But I didn't put marshmallows in it."

"Get your calculator," I told her, "and let's crunch some numbers." I began calling them out while Julie punched buttons. "One-forty for creamer. Two-forty for orange juice. One-fifty for whole milk. Three hundred in the colas. Water, zero. Strawberry wine cooler, two-fifty. Hot chocolate, no marshmallows, one-fifty."

Julie's fingers were flying on the calculator keys. When the final sum was displayed, her mouth dropped open. "I drank more than twelve hundred calories yesterday," she said in disbelief. "That's almost my total daily allowance. And I didn't chew a single one of those calories. No wonder the pounds aren't falling off."

I put my arm around my friend's shoulder. "Now that you know what's wrong, how are you going to fix it?"

"For starters, I'll study this chart and look for low-calorie alternatives for my beverages. And you can bet that from now on, I'll write everything in my diary, solid or liquid."

And that's just what she did. The big splash of coffee creamer was replaced with a small splash of skim milk. She poured skim milk rather than whole over her cereal, too. She drank no orange juice but ate an orange or half a grapefruit instead. The sugared colas were replaced with bottled water, and a four-ounce glass of dry, red wine took the place of a wine cooler. The hot chocolate was eliminated entirely.

Calories saved? More than eight hundred!

Soon Julie's body fat really did begin to melt away. By taking in no more than 1,500 calories a day—most of which she tried to consume in nutrient-dense food—and continuing with our walking program, Julie lost almost ten pounds in a month. By the time swimsuit season rolled around, she had reached her weight-loss goal of thirty-five pounds.

To celebrate, she added back some of the "forbidden" treats she missed so much, a soothing mug of hot chocolate—with marshmallows—being at the top of the list. But she is immersed in the habit of keeping a food diary, recording not only what she eats and drinks every day but also how many calories each food or beverage is worth. On the facing page of the diary, she keeps an exercise log. As long as calories consumed don't exceed calories burned, she knows she'll maintain the ideal weight she worked so hard to achieve.

And when asked what her favorite beverage is, Julie doesn't hesitate. "Water," she says. "Delicious, refreshing and zero calories!"

Jennie Ivey

The Un-Diet

Fortune and love befriend the bold.

Ovid

"No, Sue, honest, you don't look fat," my sister said.

It was the first day of my new job at a local lawn care company and I was in a panic.

"Are you sure?" I turned sideways in front of the mirror and sucked in my stomach. She had to be lying. My skirt was biting into my waistline, and I couldn't button my jacket. How had those extra pounds gotten there?

I'd always been vigilant about my weight. One careless remark when I was ten years old, "Oh, isn't she just a cute, chubby thing?" did it. I could read between the lines, f-a-t. Living in a family of skinnies, this certainly wouldn't do. And so began a lifetime of dieting. The hard-boiled egg diet took me through my preteen years and then it was on to high school with the grapefruit diet. My early career days were marked by the cabbage soup diet—much to the dismay of my coworkers. All of these kept me from being fat. But I needed to be thin. So I experimented with the Target Zone diet, Weight

Watchers and the Pyramid diet. And once I even tried fasting.

Just a few carefree months of living diet-free, like the rest of my gal pals, resulted in my present dilemma—starting my new job feeling like a blimp.

I took one last look in the mirror. Drats! The outfit needed something. I know! I quickly knotted a brightly colored scarf around my neck; let them focus on that instead of those holster hips down below. There was nothing else I could do about it now; I grabbed my keys and purse and flew out the door.

As soon as I walked into the office, my boss gave me my first task. "Here Sue, take these notes out into the warehouse and sort them by name. Each lawn specialist has their own labeled slot in the mail center." She gave me an encouraging smile and went back to typing.

I opened the door and my jaw dropped. There in front of me stood the most handsome guy I'd ever seen. His muscles rippled as he hoisted a huge bag of fertilizer over his shoulder.

I waved.

He grinned.

I felt some chemistry.

I slipped back into the office. "Who's the cute guy out there with the blond hair?"

"That's Bruce," the secretary in the corner said, "and he's dating someone."

From then on, I volunteered to do the notes each day and every other menial job that involved traipsing through "the guy area." If that meant putting up with the horrid chemical smells in the warehouse, so be it. I got to see Bruce.

I wanted to look my best for him, so every morning I was up at dawn, camouflaging those extra pounds. Black was in, prints were out, and by the time I was done primping, I almost believed I had a chance.

And one day it happened. He sauntered over as I was slipping notes into the slots.

"Hey Sue, what're you doing Friday night?" Bruce smiled and his tanned face crinkled. This gorgeous guy was really asking me out!

"I'm not sure," I tried my best to sound nonchalant. "Besides, I heard you're dating someone."

"Nah, nothing serious," he put his hand on the wall behind me, bringing us closer together.

"Well . . ." I hesitated, hoping he couldn't hear my heart thundering in my chest.

"C'mon, just burgers and a movie," he pressed, "how about it?"

"Okay," I said, feeling giddy, "sounds like fun."

We had a blast together, and he asked me out again. And again. With each date we grew closer, and within a few weeks we were an item. I was enjoying myself so much I forgot to worry about weight, exercise or that much hated four-letter word: d-i-e-t.

About a month later, Bruce came over to meet the family. It just happened to be the day my younger sister was going to the prom. She looked gorgeous as she drifted down the stairs in a swirl of peach silk, her blonde hair cascading around her shoulders. I looked at Bruce, who obviously agreed; his mouth hung open as he watched her sweep into the room.

I looked from my thin, beautiful sister to my great-looking boyfriend, and I wanted to disappear. What did he see in a chubbette like me anyway?

I pasted a smile on my face until my sister left for the dance. Then I clomped downstairs to the family room, threw myself on the sofa and bawled my eyes out.

"Hey, what's the matter?" Bruce sat next to me and

pushed my bangs back, trying to look into my eyes. "What are you crying for?"

"I-I-I'm ssssooo fat," I turned away from him. "Why are you dating me anyway? You don't belong with someone that looks like me. My sister's more your type," I blubbered.

"Sue, your sister is a real cute kid, but she's way too young for me. Besides, she's not my type—you are, and I think you're beautiful."

I turned over as tears continued to dribble down my face.

"But I have to lose this extra w-w-weight. I feel so fat and ugly-y-y-y. I don't know what you see in me." All the pain I'd experienced feeling like the chubby one in my thin, perfect family washed over me.

Bruce gathered me in his arms and just held me.

Then I felt something wet trickling down my neck. Puzzled, I pulled away and looked at Bruce. He was crying with me!

"I don't ever want to hear you call yourself fat or ugly again. No one talks that way about the woman I love, and I love you just the way you are." He leaned in and our tear-streaked faces met in a tender kiss. That was the moment I fell in love with Bruce.

Two months later, he slipped an engagement ring on my finger and on bended knee asked me to be his wife.

Dreams of a fairy-tale wedding filled my head, starting with my dress—I had to find the perfect gown. Too bad there isn't time for just one more diet, I thought longingly, but with the wedding only six months away, it wasn't possible. I visited every bridal salon within a thirty-mile radius, searching for the ideal style to flatter my fuller figure. I tried on every type of wedding dress imaginable, until I finally found it—the gown of my dreams.

"Can you wrap it up?" I asked as I gazed at the white

confection of beaded satin and delicate lace.

"Oh no, miss," she said. "We'll keep it here since you'll have to come in for several fittings between now and the wedding."

She was right. But, surprisingly, at every fitting, the seamstress had to take my gown in, not let it out. "Are you on one of those new liquid diets?" she asked as she marked the alteration with straight pins.

"No," I said. Funny, I hadn't even thought about dieting. Come to think of it, my clothes were looser lately. And I couldn't recall the last time I'd stepped on a scale.

Eight weeks later, on a perfect June day, I slipped into my wedding dress feeling radiant. I floated down the aisle thinner than I'd ever been. I beamed at my husband-to-be, waiting for me by the altar, and I knew it was all thanks to him. Bruce loved me just as I was, and that was the only diet I ever needed.

Susan A. Karas

It Takes Community

*Let's take the bouldering mistakes of the past,
And the road-blocking challenges of the present,
And build them into stairs that support our
climb into the future.*

Mattie J. T. Stepanek

Tears collected in the corners of my eyes as I crossed the threshold. They spilled down my cheeks as I unbuckled my sandals and stepped, barefoot, onto the scale. Biting my trembling lower lip, I tried to smile at the group leader's sympathetic face. I then slumped into a plastic chair next to my friend, Ursi, who had nudged me through the door. Up until now, I had always rejected community weight-loss approaches, wanting to believe I was strong enough to do this myself.

During the next half hour, I dredged up five decades' worth of tears from somewhere deep within. In those moments I wept for the little girl who prayed to be invisible as she tried on corduroys in J.C. Penney's "chubby department." I wept for the straight-A student, always chosen last for the relay team. I wept for the teenager who skipped breakfast and lunch, hoping her figure would attract a boyfriend. And I wept for the woman with expressive brown eyes who begged family photographers, "Don't shoot below the shoulders."

Struggling with my weight was nothing new. Topping 200 on the bathroom scale was nothing new. Dieting was nothing new. I was a veteran of the grapefruit juice diet, ice cream diet, high-protein diet, low-calorie diet, low-fat diet and low-carbohydrate diet, to name a few. By my fiftieth birthday I figured I had lost and gained somewhere between 500 and 1,000 pounds. What was new was acknowledging that I needed the help of others to reduce and successfully maintain the loss. That unconscious awareness was exposed to the brash light of day at that first group meeting.

Shaken, but with resolve, as well as remorse and shame, I went home that day, read the how-to booklet and started a food diary. By the second evening I was so hungry I would have eaten a piece of carpet if I'd had some good mustard to put on it. But I found that "lite" microwave popcorn was tastier and certainly better for my digestive system. The next week I went back to the meeting—four pounds lighter.

Portion control was a challenging new concept. Wasn't half a grilled chicken breast a reasonable main course? My digital kitchen scale took up permanent residence on the butcher block. With it as my new cooking companion, I discovered my "reasonable" portion weighed in at about eight ounces; a recommended entrée was only half of that. It took time to change my old habits, but after a few months I was usually content to fill only one-fourth of my dinner plate with protein and cover the rest with vegetables.

I've always taken pride in my appearance, so I highlight my hair, use good face creams, polish my toenails and color-coordinate my outfits. Why couldn't I add one more component to this picture—an average-sized body? I set out to eliminate all the Xs in my closet—the 1X, 2X and XLs on my clothing tags. Now, with the exception of an odd T-shirt that shrank in the dryer, I've done that.

My knees were also signaling me that I'd be better off thinner. At fifty-one I gave in to years of debilitating osteoarthritis pain in my left knee and had a total knee replacement. A few years later, the right knee was limping down the same path, and I was determined to avoid repeating that surgery. Carrying less weight would surely help.

When my daughter, Heather, suggested a fitness center, I balked, picturing svelte young women in fluorescent blue workout bras and shorts. But she escorted me to a gym with a sense of humor, whose slogan is "no Spandex here." She introduced me to machines I could use to build strength without compromising my joints. Maybe, just maybe, I could do this.

The pieces were beginning to mesh. I paid for my first-ever gym membership. To get me started, a personal trainer asked me a lot of questions and devised a routine for me. I wanted him to know I was also dieting, but I was ashamed to tell him where I was going for help, so I dropped my voice and whispered the name to him. Maybe he saw a glimpse of his own mother in my embarrassed face, for he replied gently, "It's okay to say it out loud." His eyes and words spoke straight to my heart, and from that day on, I did say it out loud. I started telling everyone I knew of my diet and exercise plans. They really seemed to share my joy as my success grew and my body shrank.

Two of my friends have become exercise buddies. Every Monday Ursi and I walk together along a level path overlooking Monterey Bay. At first we walked thirty minutes; she kindly slowed to my pace and stopped to rest with me on a bench midway. Now we're up to an hour nonstop, and just the other day she asked me to slow down a bit for her. On Fridays Allison and I meet at the gym, where our animated conversation makes the stationary bike wheels turn faster.

It's been nearly a year since I initiated this new lifestyle, and I'm thrilled with the results. I'm more than halfway to my goal weight and my knee pain is gone. While getting dressed one morning, I shrieked in disbelief as I pulled on a pair of jeans, zipped and snapped them, then watched them fall down around my ankles. Stepping out of the pant legs, I danced with joy around the bedroom.

My progress hasn't been rapid or easy, but it's been steady. That's probably good, because I need time to internalize all the changes. My weight has hit some plateaus—once for three months—but the inches have continued to drop, thanks to the exercise. There are days when it all seems too hard, usually when I'm overwhelmed with many other responsibilities. Then I give myself permission to "go off the wagon" for a short time. This isn't about being perfect; rather, it's about finding a way that will serve me for the long haul.

To fully savor each temporary step down in body size, I donate my clothes the minute they become loose and treat myself to an outlet shopping spree for replacements. This way there's no turning back, and I have clothes that fit and flatter without stressing the budget. And every time I lose five pounds, I buy a five-pound bag of all-purpose flour and display it on my kitchen counter. Whenever I pass my expanding collection of flour sacks, I envision all that extra bulk back on my frame. Eventually I'll give the flour to a food pantry, but for now it keeps me focused and puts a smile on my face.

I've learned that I can't do this alone, and I thrive on the encouragement of family, friends and my weight-loss group. I've always been reluctant to talk about my weight or tell anyone when I was dieting. Now I speak proudly to everyone of my efforts and goals. As a result, they become partners with me on the journey. Even the most arduous trek is more fulfilling and ultimately more successful when shared.

Pamela Wertz Peterson

Nutty Carrot Raisin Bread

MAKES 9 SERVINGS (OR 9 MUFFINS)
EACH SERVING (OR MUFFIN): 0 GRAMS SATURATED FAT

canola oil cooking spray
2 eggs, beaten
¼ cup high-oleic canola oil
¼ cup honey
¼ cup unsweetened applesauce
1 teaspoon pure vanilla extract
1 cup whole wheat flour
2 tablespoons wheat germ
¼ cup ground flaxseeds
¼ cup Splenda sugar substitute
½ teaspoon ground cloves
½ teaspoon cinnamon
½ teaspoon baking powder
½ teaspoon baking soda
1 cup shredded carrots
½ cup raisins
½ cup chopped pecans

Preheat the oven to 350°. Spray an 8½ x 4½-inch loaf pan or a 12-cup muffin tin with cooking spray.

In a small bowl, beat the eggs. Mix in the oil, honey, applesauce and vanilla extract. In a large bowl, combine the flour, wheat germ, ground flaxseeds, Splenda, ground cloves, cinnamon, baking powder and baking soda. Add the liquid ingredients to the dry ingredients and stir until well blended. Mix in the carrots, raisins and pecans.

To make bread: Pour batter into prepared pan and bake for 45 minutes. To make muffins: Pour batter into prepared muffin tin and bake for 20–25 minutes. When done, remove from pan or muffin tin and cool on a wire rack.

Reprinted from The Gold Coast Cure. ©2005 *Andrew Larson, M.D., Ivy Ingram Larson. Health Communications, Inc.*

In for a Penny, In for a Pound

Attention to health is life's greatest hindrance.

Plato

They lied to me.

They promised I'd lose ten to thirteen pounds in the first two weeks.

I didn't lose a single pound.

They said I must have been cheating.

I wasn't. Not that I haven't cheated on past diets—you know, a cookie yesterday, a bite (or two) of ice cream today—but not this time. This time I was serious.

I had tried them all. This new one was the latest in a long line of fad diets. Even my doctor lost weight on this diet. It required a strict adherence to a regimen of foods with a low glycemic index (GI). Don't ask me to explain it—something to do with how quickly carbohydrates break down in digestion. Foods with a high index were to be eliminated for the first two weeks.

Contrary to all my impulses—impulses clearly illus-trated by the size of my hips—I followed the diet's rules. No bread, rice, potatoes, pasta, baked goods—those I could understand. But fruit was also forbidden for the first two weeks. Fruit! What happened to "an apple a day keeps the doctor away"? Guess it keeps the doctor away, but not the pounds.

So there I was with my GI chart, no flour, no sugar, no fruit, not even certain vegetables with a high GI rating. But water was okay. Lots and lots of water.

It was the longest two weeks of my life. My driving motivation, besides a closetful of clothes that no longer fit, was the promise: ten to thirteen pounds in the first two weeks.

The first three days were easy. I was excited, and this particular diet was novel. After all, who ever heard of a diet that placed fruits (and some vegetables) in the same category as cookies and ice cream? In addition to the change in my eating habits, I also drank eight to ten glasses of water a day and began an exercise routine that included walking around my neighborhood every morning.

Day One: I weighed myself for an official benchmark. Ready to go!

Day Two: no change.

Day Three: still no change.

Well, I thought, *I'm less than a quarter of the way through. Maybe my body just needs to adjust.*

I drank more water.

Days Four and Five: the arrow on the scale didn't budge.

I was becoming discouraged. (Becoming? I was in a full-blown state of disappointment.) I did what most people do when they're on a diet. I talked about it. Actually, it was more whining than talking. What I could eat, what I couldn't eat. How I sloshed when I walked. Worst of all, how the bathroom scale hated me. The responses were predictable.

"Are you sure you're not cheating?" (Yes, I'm sure I'm not cheating.)

"It must be water retention." (Possibly.)

"You're not exercising enough." (Probably.)

"That's terrible. Have a chocolate kiss—you'll feel better." (That last one was from my inner child, whom I wisely chose to ignore.)

So I drank more water. Believe it or not, the best way to eliminate water retention is to drink more water. And I exercised more. Walking, bicycling, sit-ups and workout videos.

Days Six and Seven: nothing.

Day Eight: our bathroom scale owes its life to my husband. I had decided to toss it onto the curb with the rest of the household trash, but he convinced me the scale was an innocent bystander in my battle of the bulge. We'll see.

Day Nine: the arrow on the scale moved—a whole pound! Rejoice! Celebrate! Now, I was sure, the weight loss would begin in earnest. I did a little dance and broke out the celery sticks.

Day Ten: no additional movement, but that's okay. After all, I had lost a pound. Life was good.

Day Eleven: my mood matched the dark sky. The pound had returned. Why? How? I went back to my friends for advice. The consensus was that the weight was actually added muscle from the increased exercise. "Muscle weighs more than fat."

Yeah, yeah, yeah. How many times have I heard that before? Been there, done that, bought the T-shirt (in an extra-large size). I'm ready for a new destination.

Day Twelve: no change. Well, to be perfectly truthful, there was one change, but not on the scale. As a result of my daily walks around the neighborhood, I had gotten to know my neighbors, and they are really nice people. Who knew?

Day Thirteen: no change.

Day Fourteen: I didn't bother getting on the scale.

Instead, I dumped the diet book, ignored the well-meaning advice and listened to my own body. It was time to start eating a balanced diet of the foods the Creator designed it to have. Fad diets obviously weren't the answer, as my most recent experience had proven yet again.

I went shopping. I filled my cart with colorful fruits and vegetables, as well as representatives from each of the other food groups. To add fiber to my diet, "white" was out and "brown" was in, including sugar, flour and even grains such as rice. I avoided processed foods, deciding that my body didn't need to digest ingredients and chemicals that my brain couldn't pronounce.

Six months later, I've lost over twenty-five pounds. I feel better than I have in years, and I'm ready for the next twenty-five.

And I still have the same scale!

Ava Pennington

The First Day of the Best of My Life

*O*ne *of the symptoms of an approaching nervous breakdown is the belief that one's work is terribly important.*

Bertrand Russell

I smiled at the memories of the previous night's dinner. I had met some friends at one of our favorite restaurants and we'd had our regular Monday night supper of grilled double-cheese and bacon sandwiches. I savored every bite of my sandwich—determined not to miss a bit of the experience. From the sound of the crisp crust on the grilled bread to the feel of the gooey cheese to the salty sweet taste of the maple bacon, I fully enjoyed my favorite sandwich.

But that was Monday night, and it was now Tuesday morning. I bounded out of bed in the morning. I had been overweight for years. Way overweight. But things had changed. I had decided that I was tired of observing life. I wanted to be a participant, but at 260 pounds, participating was a struggle.

I made a conscious decision to begin my new lifestyle on a Tuesday. In the past, Monday had been the day I would start a diet or return to the gym. In the past, I had always ended up giving up at some point—usually by Friday. I knew that this time was different, and I was determined to start it differently.

I laughed and sang along to the radio as I drove into the office. I greeted my coworkers with a smile.

"Charmi, we need you to come over to Human Resources."

I smiled as I made my way across the building. I was due for a raise and had just worked myself silly on an international project. I hadn't expected the recognition to come that quickly but I was happy that I was going to be rewarded for my efforts. And what a day for it to happen!

"Sit down, please."

I looked into the face of the HR representative and continued to smile. Finally, payoff!

"Charmi, there's no easy way to say this, so I'm not going to beat around the bush. We're letting you go."

It wasn't until later that I could actually recall what the HR representative had said during the rest of our meeting. My mind took in what my heart couldn't hear at the time. I walked back to my desk, retrieved my purse and left the building. The first day of the "best" of my life had taken a sudden turn in an unexpected direction.

I don't remember driving home. I don't remember changing out of my business suit. I don't remember a thing between leaving the office and standing in front of my TV. Much to my surprise, I found myself standing there in the living room watching the start of my new exercise video. I glanced over my shoulder toward the kitchen, and in that moment I made the decision of my life. I turned back toward the television and began moving to the music. The sweat pouring from my face mixed with angry and confused tears. When the video was over, I sat on the floor and cried some more.

With that one simple decision to exercise rather than get something to eat, I took full control of my future. As the days wore on, I held fast to my decision to honor myself by honoring my new lifestyle. Maybe I did it out of desperation—it was the only thing that I felt I had any control over in my life. Maybe I did it out of fear—what if I couldn't get a new job because of my weight? In the end, all that mattered was that I did do it. More importantly, that I chose to do it.

There were several ups and downs—both emotionally and on the scale—over the next sixteen months. But in less than a year and a half, I had moved back to my home-town, found a fabulous job and had lost 127 pounds.

That was several years ago. Since then I've changed jobs a few times, moved twice and have gained weight. A lot of weight. I woke up one morning not too long ago and found myself back where I had been, both physically and mentally, on that Tuesday many years before. I pulled out my exercise videos and got them ready for when I got home from work

After a very healthy breakfast, I headed for work with a renewed attitude. Shortly after lunch, HR made an announcement.

"We will be experiencing staff reductions over the next few weeks."

I couldn't help it, I had to laugh. That announcement—and its timing—let me know that good things lay ahead.

Charmi Schroeder

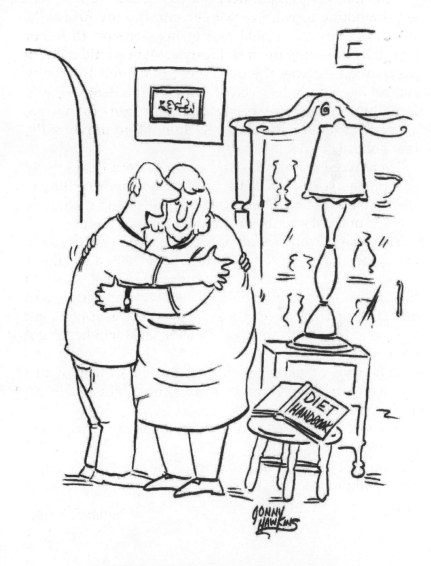

"Is there any way you can lose weight
without having any less to hug?"

Reprinted with permission of Jonny Hawkins.

5

THE
NEW YOU

If one advances confidently in the direction of his dreams, and endeavors to live the life which he has imagined, he will meet with success unexpected in common hours.

Henry David Thoreau

Fabulously Fighting Fit at Fifty
(and Beyond)

I don't know what the big deal is about old age.
Old people who shine from the inside look ten to
twenty years younger.

Dolly Parton

I was approaching one of life's major milestones—my fiftieth birthday. I was also fast approaching another peak in my roller coaster–style weight management plan that had been a part of my life for as long as I can remember. So what better occasion than to make some serious lifestyle changes and lose some weight? I had spent years setting goals for myself, reaching them, feeling great and then reverting back to all the bad habits that got me onto the slippery slope of weight gain in the first place. I tried all the various diets that came and went as medical and marketing opinions changed. I counted fat, fiber, calories and ounces and always lost weight. What I never managed to achieve was a state of maintenance, until now.

One day my friend Carol said, "How about doing a personal training program together?" I thought, *You must be joking,* but I said, "Okay, I'll give it a go," trying to sound positive. This was the most important step I have ever taken into the weight-loss arena. Carol and I undertook a twelve-week program, which consisted of three days a week weight training and three days a week cardio workouts with Mark, a qualified trainer at Fighting Fit Academy. I had been used to exercising and was reasonably fit. Over the years I had donned Lycra and embraced all the latest exercise trends. However, I had a feeling this would be a serious challenge, and I was not wrong.

Arriving at the gym on the first day, I was excited, but scared. We were weighed and measured; then Mark explained the program to us. I could not believe the weight I was expected to lift, press and carry, but "can't" was a word Mark did not permit in his gym, so finding the power and strength needed, I did what I was told.

After the first day I was tired but elated, and I slept well after a long soak in a bath filled with Epsom salts and aromatherapy oils. The next day I could not move, walking was nearly impossible and areas of my body hurt where I did not know I had muscles. The next two weeks were more of the same, and I was constantly sore and tired. However, I gradually became stronger, found the training easier and recovered faster. I also began to feel invigorated instead of tired.

In parallel with the training program, I was introduced to a different way of eating—not a diet, but a sensible eating plan designed to provide the energy and nutrition needed for strenuous exercise and also designed for weight loss. I no longer ate a big meal at night but instead ate small meals, six times a day, including some protein with each meal, and greatly reduced my overall carbohydrate intake. I was rarely hungry, and what is more, I felt great. I had one day a week when I could eat what I wanted, but just knowing that I could do so provided an escape hatch that I actually did not take advantage of very often.

I had expected overnight changes, but this program was not about a quick fix. It took six weeks before anything happened, and then my shape began to change. At the end of the program, I was astounded at the results. I had lost a little more than fifteen pounds, which may not seem like a lot of weight, but by converting fat to toned muscle, I had lost inches in all the important places, rediscovered my waist and found that my small frame was quite shapely after all. I was ecstatic and basked in this feeling, soaking up compliments and enjoying the gasps of amazement at my "before and after" photos.

I had reached a pinnacle of achievement, but the real challenge was just beginning. This was not about reaching a goal and then stopping but was the start of a new lifestyle. If I was to find my Holy Grail of maintenance, I needed to make a major mind shift. I always remember one of my diet program leaders saying that the most important area for weight loss is the top three inches of our head, and that the rest follows.

I have had to acknowledge that life is not fair. I will never be able to eat what I want without getting fat, and I will always need lots of physical activity, so for the first time I accepted this as my new philosophy and turned away from the path of striving toward a goal paved with sacrifice and denial. Instead I have extended the timeframe of this goal into a lifelong journey to be cherished and enjoyed.

Now I exercise daily and eat sensibly and moderately most of the time, but I do give myself permission to indulge in the occasional treat. In this way my weight has stabilized. I never allow it to fluctuate by more than five pounds at a time.

I use my own body signals to recognize when my intake

(food) and output (exercise) is out of balance and correct the imbalance immediately. I also know that the feel-good factor from a good workout is far more satisfying and longer lasting that the ephemeral joy of tantalizing the taste buds. I took up bike riding, yoga and tai chi, all of which has helped me feel in control of my body, disperse stress before it builds up and divert extreme emotions so that I can handle them better.

Two years later, I have maintained my weight and exercise regime, and I have found that I can easily cope with the changes that are a natural, but difficult, part of life for a woman in her fifties. I maintain my sanity by continuing the path I started with lots of invigorating and varied exercise. I took that first step and began to experience a feeling of well-being. Before long, my motivation led me to a new and exciting place. Now nothing can hold me back.

Janet Marianne Jackson

A Second Chance at Life

*If you can't be a good example, then you'll just
have to be a horrible warning.*

Catherine Aird

Set a goal, follow the course and you achieve your
dream. Sounds easy, doesn't it?

Over a number of years I've gained five pounds here
and another five pounds there; all of it seemed to settle
between my waist and my knees. *Part of getting older,* I told
myself. *I could lose this weight,* I thought. I did exactly that
. . . many times. Whenever I quit dieting, back it came,
along with a few more pounds. I finally hit on the perfect
rationalization. The only way to keep this weight off is to
diet for the rest of my life, and I'm not willing to do that—
perfect reasoning for someone who loves to eat and enjoys
cooking and baking. My goal was too tough to achieve. I
dismissed it with a shrug and continued eating the good
things I craved.

Then my husband, Ken, threw a curveball at me. The
man who had low blood pressure, low cholesterol, was
Mr. Easygoing and only a few pounds overweight had a

heart attack on the golf course one clear February day. Golf buddies rushed him to the clubhouse and called an ambulance. Off he went to the emergency room where he was stabilized and transferred to a tiny little helicopter for a fifty-mile flight to our state capital and a larger hospital. By the time I arrived at the hospital, the cardiologist had performed a heart catheterization followed by angioplasty. He implanted a stent into the main artery of Ken's heart when this critical artery showed a 99-percent blockage. Ken came ever so close to not making it. Needless to say, many prayers of thanksgiving were offered by me, by our family and our friends, and by the patient, too. After a short hospital stay, the cardiologist dismissed him with instructions for a brand-new lifestyle.

Diet and exercise became the key words in our vocabulary from that day on. Our goal? Simply that we both live a long and full life. To do that, we had to change our way of eating, our exercise habits and our attitudes. Easy enough to do, we thought, when living is the prize. I'd been given the diet instructions, which turned out to be pretty simple. Think low-fat. Think low-cholesterol. Most important of all . . . have small portions of all things, always!

I subscribed to magazines with light recipes, checked out low-fat cooking Web sites and spent time revising old-favorite recipes. I filled our plates with far less food than ever before, remembering how the doctor had emphasized the importance of small portions. I baked only occasionally and used canola oil instead of butter when I made cookies or muffins. At restaurants, we ate half of what we ordered and brought the rest home. The whole new lifestyle was easier than I'd feared. I could ignore a grumble or two from Ken about how I was starving him.

And then, the first distraction arose. We hesitated, and we slipped back a little bit when we were invited out to dinner. There before us lay a table laden with forbidden foods and a hostess urging us to fill our plates and have seconds. I suddenly had a brief glimpse into what Adam and Eve must have felt in the garden. We ate more than we should have, and we felt miserable. Our stomachs were no longer accustomed to such rich food. At home, and back on track once again, we continued on the pre-scribed diet—fruit in place of cookies and cake, carrot and celery sticks instead of chips, four ounces of steak rather than eight. The longer we practiced the diet, the easier it became. The pounds we shed encouraged us to keep going.

Another distraction slowed us down. This time we were tripped up by a three-week vacation on a river cruiser. Meals were gourmet offerings, including lavish buffets, scrumptious desserts and delicious breads. No doubt about it. We ate far less than most of the other passengers, but we also ate far more than we had been doing at home. We continued to exercise daily, and when we arrived back home, we went right back on the program.

Yes, we slide occasionally, but only a little, and over four years later our new lifestyle has turned into a habit. Ken has lost forty pounds, and I shed twenty-eight. We're both down to our college weight, and we feel great. Maybe a distraction will slow us now and then, but we won't col-lapse in a heap and shed tears. No, we'll keep taking care of ourselves: today, tomorrow and forever.

Nancy Julien Kopp

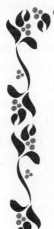

Oven-Steamed Asian-Style Fish

MAKES 4 SERVINGS
EACH SERVING: 43 GRAMS PROTEIN, TRACE CARBOHYDRATE

4 six-ounce thick fish fillets (halibut, salmon, swordfish,
    red snapper, cod or sea bass)
2 cups sliced brown or white mushrooms
2 tablespoons low-sodium tamari soy sauce
2 tablespoons dry sherry
1 tablespoon pure-pressed sesame oil
1 tablespoon fresh lime juice
⅓ cup chopped fresh scallions
1 tablespoon chopped fresh mint
2 tablespoons chopped fresh cilantro
2 minced garlic gloves
2 teaspoons peeled and finely minced fresh ginger
cayenne pepper, to taste
1 lime cut into wedges, for garnish
4 fresh cilantro sprigs, for garnish

    Rinse fish under cold water and pat dry with
paper towels. Arrange fish fillets in a greased baking dish. Top with sliced mushrooms. In a small
bowl, combine soy sauce, sherry, sesame oil, lime
juice, scallions, mint, cilantro, garlic and ginger.
Season to taste with cayenne pepper. Pour over
fish and marinate at least 30 minutes.
    Preheat oven to 375°. Bake, covered with foil,
until fish turns opaque and flakes easily with a
fork, about 20 minutes. Garnish with fresh lime
wedges and cilantro sprigs and serve immediately.

Reprinted from The Schwarzbein Principle Cookbook. ©1999
Diana Schwarzbein, M.D., Nancy Deville and Evelyn Jacob.
Health Communications, Inc.

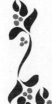

A Soul-Searching, Pound-Shedding Vacation

The person who removes a mountain begins by carrying away small stones.

Author Unknown

I was cruising 3,000 feet in the air, over the burnt sunset-hued Grand Canyon, tucked comfortably in a window seat (albeit economy) when it hit me—I was heading to Los Cabos, Mexico, for a once-in-a-lifetime splurge of a vacation, and I was not the tiniest bit excited. Instead of palm trees, lazy morning breakfasts and endless ocean images clouding my thoughts, I was thinking about one and only one thing—the way my out-of-shape, overweight body would look in a swimsuit that had been bought four months ago for what I wrongly assumed would be a leaner, healthier me.

As it turns out, the vacation planning that was supposed to spur my weight-loss regimen did just the opposite. I saved extra spending money by skipping my weekly yoga classes. I cut back on exercising to work overtime in preparation for a week off of work, and last-minute packing stress had led to massive overeating in the three days beforehand. The bottom line: my bikini was one size smaller than the normal me and I was likely one size larger.

It didn't take long for my fiancé to realize that a tear had slid down my cheek. He looked at me in astonishment, obviously wondering what on earth could be wrong—we had been waiting and planning for this day for months.

He must have gathered the words "swimsuit," "me" and "body" from my nondescript mumbles, because his response was a simple (but genuine), "I was wondering where all that ice cream went!" Then he continued with a more thoughtful approach.

"Well, let's use this vacation to do something about it. No excuses," his voice was helpful, but a stern undertone told me that my weight- and eating-related issues were wearing him thin (ironically enough).

I thought for a moment. Spend my vacation trying to get back on track? My vacation? This was supposed to be a break from the everyday monotony of diet, work and exercise. But wait, I suppose that I hadn't kept up on that at home either.

I decided then and there that my new motto would be "no excuses." If there was one thing that was simply in-escapable, it was the importance of healthy living. Despite my weakness for sugary treats and carbohydrate-laden snacks, I knew that what I wanted most was a healthy body. I grabbed a pen and notepad and got to work on the flight—not a minute more would be wasted. I jotted down my goals (both realistic and dream ones), the ways that I would achieve them, the sacrifices that I would make and the excuses that I would not.

Four hours and ten notepad-scribbled pages later, I had a plan. A good, solid plan. And then I did something that in all of my dieting obstacles I'd never done . . . I handed the notebook to my fiancé and asked him to help hold me accountable. The fact that I was allowing him into this issue that shook my insecurities to the core was a huge step—for myself and our relationship. Not only did he promise to give it his utmost attention, he appreciated the opportunity to contribute to my livelihood in such a way. We spent the rest of the plane ride brainstorming healthy eating and fitness ideas. By the time flight #0292 had landed, I felt I had a new lease on life. Los Cabos was welcoming a new, updated me.

Mornings were started with fresh, low-fat breakfasts, snacks were healthy and light. We ate early evening dinners, accompanied by an occasional glass of celebratory wine. Finding a local yoga class was as easy as asking the concierge, and we filled our afternoons with side trips that provided good workouts in disguise—kayaking, swimming, long walks and bike rentals.

By the trip's end I had lost five pounds, but more importantly, I felt good. It was easy to slip into my swimsuit when I knew that I'd spent the day working for the good of my body.

My initial tears of frustration had triggered something inside of me, and I'd no longer wait for a vacation to change myself for the better. As a protection plan for our own well-being, we booked our hotel for another week on the exact same dates the following year. This time around there would be no excuses and no reason to spoil the excitement of our romantic, adventurous rendezvous. Because when it comes right down to it, a body needs healthy fuel, physical work and determination, whether you're at home in suburban Chicago or on the emerald and turquoise waters of Los Cabos, happily baking in the sun—in a perfectly fitted bikini, of course.

Jessica Blaire

7 Hints for Navigating
Your Local Supermarket

First, the good news: you finally made a commitment to eating healthily. And the bad news? Those old temptations haven't gone anywhere. How in the world can you make grocery shopping a kinder, gentler experience for your waistline? As someone who recently reached her own personal weight-loss goal, here are my tips for surviving and thriving while doing food shopping.

Try incorporating even just a few of these tips and pretty soon the grocery store will be your friend again, and not your weight-loss foe. Happy, healthy shopping!

Know where you're going. Focus your efforts in these areas: dairy, produce, deli/meat and frozen food. Choose low-fat options when possible, and avoid preprepared foods, which tend to be fried or laden with extra salt and/or heavy sauces. Stock up on fruits and veggies, and go for the pre-packaged varieties if it will help you get your daily allotment.

Proceed to other aisles with caution. Don't go up and down each and every one. Just hit the ones you need. Or to put it another way, if cookies call your name, steer clear of them.

Size matters. Can you just eat one? If not, that megasized container may spell disaster for your waistline no matter how much money you might save. If you can't trust yourself to control portions, let someone else do the work for you. Many supermarket items come in single-serving packages to make portion control simpler. Just remember to only eat one portion at a sitting—not the whole box.

Just say no . . . to samples. Mindless eating inevitably leads to weight gain. How many of those mini-corn dogs did you have anyway? Was it three or was it four? And what exactly was in those things anyway? If you're committed to watching your calories, then just pass up those freebies. This leads us to the cardinal rule. . . .

Don't shop when you're hungry. I would also stretch this rule to say don't go food shopping when you're stressed or upset either. I'm no Pollyanna, so I know that isn't always possible. If you think you might be feeling munchy, have something to eat before you leave home or keep a healthy snack available to tide you over. Don't rely on food to soothe you either. Plan another way to "reward" yourself, whether it's a bubble bath, a walk or just listening to your favorite music. Maybe those cookies or chips will temporarily make you feel better, but how will you feel when your clothes are tight once again?

Go fishing for condiments. Being virtuous and eating healthy is hard, not to mention sometimes boring. So load up on healthy dips. Three great choices are salsa, hummus and bean dip. My personal favorite is adding fat-free whipped topping to fruit, especially berries. If you want a little heat, try adding salsa, hot sauce, horseradish and specialty mustards to your food. Don't forget that lower-fat sour cream, salad dressings and yogurts can all be the starting points for some fabulous dips. Go a step further and make spices your friend. From mild to wild, they make foods from veggies to breads to meats more fun.

Don't pull the "trigger." In my family, carbs are our trigger foods—bread, potatoes, pasta, we love 'em all. Decide whether you just have to give them up totally or if you can benefit by small changes. For example, if you love french fries, you could decide that you will only have them as a special treat, or maybe you can substitute healthier versions, such as baked ones from the frozen food section, or make your own using sweet potatoes. If that doesn't work, try avoiding the trigger food for two weeks. You could pretend that your grocery store is all out of them and the next shipment won't arrive until then. After fourteen days, reassess. You might surprise yourself and find you've lost the craving for it completely.

Tricia Finch

Monday Morning Blues

Tell me what you eat, and I shall tell you what you are.

Anthelme Brillat-Savarin

My right hand dug deeper into the bag of chocolates, again! There I was, first thing Monday morning, breaking the promise I'd made the night before. I'd promised myself there'd be no more drowning my woes in a pound of chocolates or an entire loaf of hot, crusty bread. But by midmorning I'd consumed half of the bag of chocolates and had begun to devour a loaf of hot sourdough French bread, one slice after another, thickly spread with pure creamery butter.

It was amazing how I rationalized my behavior. I blamed it all on stress. After all, a large conglomerate had gobbled up my employer of twenty years, there'd been a reduction in salary and benefits, and I was subjected to longer work hours. And I continued to overindulge in food, which at the end of the day only made me fatter, not happier.

After six months of helping make the merger a smooth

transition, I announced my retirement. After a magnificent retirement send-off, my husband and I purchased a condo where we'd always planned to retire, the central coast of California. Although I was retiring ten years earlier than planned, my husband assured me I had made the right decision. "You can finally do what you've always wanted to do, live near the ocean and write full-time."

I settled into the new community and made many new friends, most of them writers like myself. I thrived on being among my peers. I was overjoyed at the writing opportunities that came my way. Life was good. In the back of my mind lingered the nagging question: why was I still gorging myself with food? I even ignored my doctor's concern about my weight and reasons for lowering my cholesterol.

I was eating when I was glad and when I was sad; I was running out of excuses. I could no longer zip my favorite black slacks, and to my dismay they did not come in any larger size. That very Sunday evening I vowed to seek help on Monday morning. I'd follow my doctor's advice and sign up for weight counseling.

My knees shook when I approached the counter to register for weight counseling, but I felt at ease when a gentleman with a smiling face greeted me, "Welcome, I'm one of the weight counselors here. My name is Frank."

I fought back the tears as I introduced myself and confessed to him how desperate I felt. As I filled out the paperwork, Frank uttered softly, "As of today, desperation and self-loathing are banished from your vocabulary."

Next, it was time to step on the scales. I didn't want to look, but I had to face the awful truth; I had gained forty pounds. I felt my cheeks grow hot, I closed my eyes, but that didn't stop the tears from trickling down my red face.

"You have to think of this as a lifestyle change, not a diet," Frank said, as he handed me a tissue. "This program is not a quick fix. Once you lose the weight you cannot go back to your old habits, and you won't want to."

My lifestyle change entailed banishing my two addictions, chocolate and white bread, from the house. Breakfast would no longer consist of chocolate candy and a cup of coffee. Actually, I'd forgotten I really liked cereal with fresh strawberries for breakfast.

The first week I lost three pounds. "So, during your first week did you have any problems getting used to eating healthy again?" Frank asked. I grumbled that keeping a journal of every morsel I put in my mouth was time-consuming. Frank chuckled and replied, "When you nibble, you gotta scribble. It's the only way I've been able to keep my eighty pounds off for the past fifteen years."

I never complained again and faithfully wrote in my journal every day. I continued to lose weight, but it was a slow process. Frank's words kept me from getting discouraged. "Remember, set your goal weight at something you can live with. When you look at the weight range for your age, be realistic; don't beat yourself up because you can't fit into the size you wore when you were a teenager."

I learned how to eat healthy; I was no longer a member of the clean-your-plate club. My exercise of choice was walking, and it worked. At the end of six months, I will never forget hearing Frank's exclamation, "Congratulations! You've lost 42.6 pounds! You've reached your goal!"

It has been two and a half years, and I am still under my goal weight. I will admit there are days that I struggle, but food is no longer my security blanket. I've kept my promise—no more Monday morning blues for me!

Georgia A. Hubley

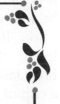

Roasted Summer Squash Combo

MAKES 4 SERVINGS
EACH SERVING: 0 GRAMS SATURATED FAT

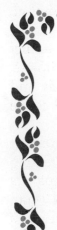

2 tablespoons extra virgin olive oil
1 tablespoon crushed garlic
1 teaspoon dried rosemary
2 medium zucchini, cut lengthwise into ½-inch-thick
  slices
2 medium yellow summer squash, cut lengthwise into
  ½-inch-thick slices
2 red onions, cut crosswise into ½-inch-thick slices
Salt, to taste
White pepper, to taste
¼ cup balsamic vinegar, or less, to taste

Preheat oven to 450°. In a small bowl, stir together the olive oil, crushed garlic and rosemary.

Line a large cookie sheet with aluminum foil and arrange vegetables evenly on the foil. Drizzle the oil over the vegetables and toss to coat. Season vegetables to taste with salt and white pepper. Transfer vegetables to the oven and roast for 20 minutes.

Remove vegetables from the oven and drizzle with balsamic vinegar to taste. Serve immediately or at room temperature.

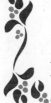

Reprinted from Fitter, Firmer, Faster. ©*2006 Andrew Larson, M.D., Ivy Ingram Larson. Health Communications, Inc.*

My Last Twenty Pounds

Life is a tragedy for those who feel, and a comedy for those who think.

Jean de la Bruyère

My last twenty pounds and I have a part-time relationship. Ten of those pounds are a group of homebodies. They wave off their more mobile relatives and stay firmly put. The other ten leave for the summer, but as winter approaches they must think of the family they left on my belly because they come back home for the holidays. I watch their comings and goings confident that, when all of us are ready, we'll never see each other again.

I've lost another forty pounds permanently. It took two years for them to go, but we parted as friends. It wasn't always easy giving up the protection they provided.

For most of my life I have been embarrassed by emotions. I thought that there was a difference between how I felt and how I was supposed to feel. Good people, I thought, didn't get so angry, unhappy or whatever this new feeling cute boys inspired was. By my early teens I was twenty pounds overweight, to buffer the space between my embarrassment and the world of slow dancing and kissing.

That buffer was not enough as my feelings became complicated with artistic passion, real romantic desires, a sense of dissatisfaction and a mysterious inadequacy in the face of love. The more complex and unfathomable my feelings became, the more I sought to numb them.

As adulthood progressed, I numbed my emotions by strengthening my five physical senses. Here was a wealth of experience I could understand through eating. The visual changes in the patina of crust as dough bakes into bread. The aromatic bouquet of red wine as it breathes. There was also the musical sizzle of butter browning in the pan. And taste. Everything has one taste as it crosses the lips, another on the tongue as it is transferred to the teeth for chewing and still another as it travels down the throat. Perhaps surprisingly, since I had gained another twenty pounds, this was also a highly sexual time in my life. The satisfaction my senses brought me through food, drink and sex replaced the shame of dealing with depths of feeling and the realities of intimate connection.

The world of the senses did not protect me. My so-called romances brought disruption. I developed a fear of being alone. I was worried I would be seen as a stereotypical fat girl, unworthy of love or acceptance. There were loud arguments that I knew would turn violent if I didn't stop them through some gesture of self-abasement. During this time, I abandoned my sensuality and sought the comforts of fullness. I did not care what I ate. I did not care how it was prepared or if it was quality food. During this great emptiness, I gained twenty more pounds.

Then I got smart. Suddenly, I started talking to people about what I was feeling. I realized I had to take care of my emotions and the information they were giving me. To learn to feel, I discovered, was to learn to communicate and to make lasting connections. I did not join a gym and find true love there. I did not discover a magic formula to erase years of poor eating habits and a tendency to over-indulge. I did not become an ascetic subsisting on leaves and water.

Instead, I discovered there was some essence in me that I shared with every other human being on the planet. Sharing my own feelings with the people I met and listening to their experiences was enlightening. I began to live with my sensuality rather than for sensual experience. I no longer believed that I was fundamentally different, and I stopped being embarrassed by my own emotions. I believe that the first twenty pounds came off through the release of that heavy burden.

The second twenty pounds were a practical and methodical loss. The many options of lifestyle change were often overwhelming when I needed to focus on coming out of numbness. Simplicity worked for me. I learned that frozen vegetables are the working person's best friends in the kitchen. They are inexpensive, quickly prepared, and come in a huge variety of flavors and colors. I learned to exercise every day, even if it is only ten minutes of stretching. It helps to ease stress and frustration. I stopped watching television after 9:00 PM. It made me feel inadequate with my physical imperfections and then tempted me with fast-food commercials.

The last twenty pounds and I are still figuring things out. They make their occasional forays out into the world, and I learn gently how to experience life without them. It's a new emotion, but I'm finally open to feeling it.

Kate Baggott

Setting Goals and Reaping Rewards

When I talk about my weight loss to people who have never had a significant weight problem, I tell them that I did not see reality in the mirror. Sure, I knew what the scale said and what size I wore, but before losing seventy-five pounds, I only saw what I thought were my positive attributes when I saw my reflection. I saw fabulous hair, expressive eyes, youthful skin and a pretty face. I didn't see what 225 pounds really looked like on a 5'2" frame. My brain, in denial, didn't let me see my fat.

I realized I was truly obese when I overheard another therapist at the clinic where I teach children with learning disabilities tell a parent, "Your son's teacher will be the heavyset woman in the staff picture." I had taken a picture with several colleagues, and the picture was framed and put in the lobby where I worked. There were four fit women, and then there was me. On a day when I thought I looked my best, I photographed as a fat, frumpy, middle-aged woman. I was devastated.

Having never been successful with a diet because I never truly thought I needed one, I didn't know where to start, so I just stopped eating. For a month, I lived on salad, diet soda and anything with zero calories, especially zero-calorie gum and hard candies. I bought a scale and saw "225" staring back at me, but with this semistarvation diet, I saw no change. I told a friend about my diet and the frustration of not losing. Her reaction was, "That's because your body is in starvation mode. You have to eat or it stores fat." She said she ate five or six small meals a day, was never hungry, and unless she binged, she kept her weight down.

It's often difficult to take diet advice from a thin person, but I knew my friend understood nutrition. Knowing my eating habits, she suggested Atkins. I bought the book and my husband and I decided we could be happy with this change of eating for the long term. We decided that this couldn't just be a quick diet and then back to bad habits; we would have to change our eating habits forever. Atkins was not a difficult diet to follow, and within days of starting a low-carbohydrate lifestyle, we began to see the scale move downward.

As an educational therapist, I had the added advantage of knowing what setting goals and receiving rewards does for children who see what appear to be insurmountable problems. I have often used goal setting and rewards to help them achieve more than they thought they could. I decided I needed the same motivation to keep me on track. I kept a chart for myself and my husband and posted it on the mirror in our bathroom. On it, we wrote our weight and measurements. On mine, I also listed my goals and the rewards. Crossing off each one was also a reward in itself.

My goals were very simple and fun. When I lost ten pounds, I made my hair lighter. When I lost ten more, I got my ears pierced. When I was down thirty pounds, I added more holes in my ears. I told my coworkers, friends and family about these, and when I had something new, such as a third hole in each ear, the reaction was a positive, "How much have you lost? I see you rewarded yourself!" There were additional goals. I had a red suede jacket that I had bought years earlier and quickly grew out of. When I fit into it again, I went out and bought a smaller black suede jacket for a lot less money because I didn't have to buy it in a specialty store for large women.

I had set up goals like weighing less than my husband and fitting into a pair of tight white jeans like the ones I was wearing when I met him. As with most weight loss, the early pounds are the easiest. As time goes on, there is still loss, but the amounts tend to be less. Getting rewards for goals made the potential frustration seem more attainable. Throughout the last year, I've mentioned to people that when I lost seventy-five pounds, I was going to cut my hair short. For years, I hid behind a long mane of hair, which I thought hid my size. In fact, it was a security blanket of sorts. It hid nothing.

Several weeks ago, I had it all chopped off. Snip. Snip. Snip. Over two feet of hair fell to the floor. The reaction from almost everyone was that I looked great and YOUNGER. When I got on the scale after my haircut, I weighed two pounds less, too! Of course, I lost two pounds of hair! I've even dyed my hair back to its natural color, knowing now that I need no more disguises or security blankets.

I also no longer need rewards. I have another twenty-five pounds to go, and the reward now is the weight loss and the knowledge of how much control I have taken of my body, my life and myself. That's the greatest reward of all.

Felice Prager

No More Pancakes on This Woman's Shopping List!

The family is one of nature's masterpieces.

George Santayana

Everybody in our family looks forward to Saturdays. Nobody has to think about work or school. We sleep late. Even Tobby, our cocker spaniel mix, appreciates that.

All families accumulate traditions, large and small. It has been a Saturday tradition in our family to sit around the breakfast table together and dig into pancakes made from a packaged mix. We're not all maple syrup fans, but we each have our own pancake ideas. Some of us prefer pancakes topped with powdered sugar, others with a dab of strawberry jam, others with sliced peaches. Over the years, we've experimented with all varieties of pancake possibilities.

Toby takes his pancake plain, cut into a dozen or so pieces, in his dog bowl. Toby is so enthusiastic about our Saturday breakfast routine that we call him our Pancake Prince. Every Saturday for six years, Toby has practiced, if not perfected, his pancake habit.

Turning over a new leaf, the day came that two human members of the family were about to turn forty. Call it a midlife crisis if you must, but they decided to adopt a healthier lifestyle and shed a few of those extra pounds around the middle. The result was that two parents and four teens got involved in sports of all sorts—basketball, soccer, even in-line skating. Saturdays were no longer the same. The pancake griddle was retired to the back of an upper cupboard. Instead of lounging in bed for extra hours on Saturday, we all got up about 8:00 AM to go for a brisk walk with Toby. Over time, the distances increased. That is to say, a few blocks in spring became a few miles by fall. Except for the first weeks, nobody seemed to mind the exercise.

Toby continued to check his bowl for something special, but there were no more Saturday pancakes to be seen in our house. No pancakes with butter, no pancakes smothered in whipped cream. The humans were eating (and enjoying) fresh fruits and dry toast, maybe some plain cereal. That was the extent of the Saturday breakfast gala. It was indistinguishable from a workday routine. We talked about what foods we bought and we talked about what we ate. Shopping lists no longer mentioned pancakes, and the kitchen table had healthy food on it seven days a week.

Nobody dared discuss the good old pancake days, perhaps fearing the very mention might somehow invite invisible calories. It wasn't just the humans who lost weight, of course. Toby, no longer being the resident Pancake Prince, also took on a leaner shape.

Another lifestyle change for us meant almost no snacking, so Toby could no longer expect to be treated to a peanut or pretzel when the family was watching television. Watching television? Who had time for that anymore? With baseball season and swimming, followed by soccer and then all the half-marathons, it was just about time for football (and maybe a little leaf raking around the yard). Could we find time for some serious ice skating before it was time to shovel snow? The entire calendar had become very active indeed!

The crowning moment came about two years post-pancake. Toby had the vet's permission to accompany two of the kids walking a half-marathon. By then it seemed as if they'd been in training for what seemed a lifetime. The former Pancake Prince and his human pals got cheered along the entire route. Nobody doubted the trim trio clinched the blue ribbon for best of show that day!

Roberta Beach Jacobson

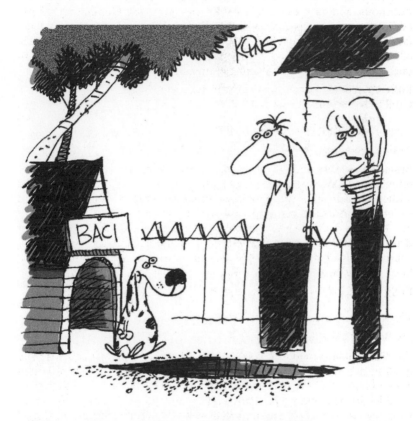

"The tunnel starts from under the fridge and leads to this hole that was under his dog house. The mystery why we have a fat dog is solved."

Reprinted by permission of Jerry King.

Beating the Genes

Nobody's family can hang out the sign, "Nothing the matter here."

Chinese proverb

"Are you carbohydrate sensitive?" my gynecologist asked. I'd asked for thyroid tests because I'd been rapidly gaining weight. Carbohydrate sensitive? Was this something like being lactose intolerant? I liked carbs. Carbs liked me. So what? My tests came back fine, but the weight question remained unanswered. I felt there was something more here.

Fast-forward five years after that carb question. My carbohydrate knowledge amounted to what the media fed us: that thousands of people were jumping on the Atkins low-carb diet. Me? I hated diets.

At my next appointment, my 5'4" frame weighed in at a whopping 201 pounds. Chills ran down my spine, kindling an unfamiliar fear. Just a year before, my fifty-two-year-old mother died on my thirtieth birthday, and she hadn't even been sick! Her death devastated our family. In hindsight, she harbored many health risks: obesity, untreated high blood pressure, an enlarged heart from childhood rheumatic fever, a maternal grandmother who suffered several strokes before age seventy and a maternal grandfather who had two heart bypass surgeries before age seventy.

It's apparent now that our family was naive about these health risks that cut Mom's life short. The doctor blamed her death on pulmonary embolism. The coroner said, "heart attack." Regardless of the cause, multiple warning signs were present, but ignored.

I was horrified to see the scale read 201. If the above warning signs weren't enough to scare me, diabetes ran on both sides of the family as well. I suddenly felt that I was up to bat in the ninth inning of the World Series and down in the count by two strikes. My situation weighed heavily on me, both figuratively and literally.

What were my chances of beating the odds stacked against me? After that appointment, I started viewing my life as things being IN or OUT of my control. Period. Genetics, obviously, were "out." But if I didn't get a handle on things in my control, I could repeat a sad history if I died young, like Mom.

What I ate was in my control, so I began analyzing meals. Monday: pasta, bread. Tuesday: meat, potatoes, rolls (gobs of butter!). Wednesday: take-out. Thursday: goulash. Friday: take-out—again.

My diet could've been a promo for "Carbs-R-Us." At that moment, I decided my family would not endure heartbreak, as I had in losing Mom so soon. I vowed to cut back on pasta, potatoes, bread, sweets and inactivity.

I learned the difference between "good" and "bad" carbs, and that our bodies actually need good carbs to function correctly. I also learned that serotonin is a chemical in our brains responsible for making us happy. When serotonin levels are low, we feel unhappy. I'm not a scientist, but now I understand that high-carb foods feed the brain's serotonin levels. As I ingested high-carb foods, I increased the levels in my brain that were low to begin with. My brain liked it and craved more. My body chemistry was actually partly to blame for my cravings!

I started making healthier choices at the grocery store. I cooked similar meals, but with healthier alternatives. I paid attention to portion sizes, often reducing them. Fruits and nuts became standard snacks instead of chocolate. And water—lots of water—replaced soda. My weight dropped significantly. Eventually I stopped eating starchy foods completely and reduced my sugar intake. It wasn't that I couldn't eat them, I simply didn't want them. For the first time, it was working for me!

Nine months later, sixty pounds lighter, five sizes smaller, feeling good and looking great, I joined a fitness gym. My personal trainer taught me to lift weights three days a week and walk on the other days. And surprisingly, I loved it! Muscles appeared out of nowhere. Inches disappeared.

Empowered is now a common word in my vocabulary. I am thrilled with the way I now look and feel. The mirror, once foe, is now my friend. I like what I see. Most importantly, I like who I see. A strong, confident mother, wife and woman; a woman I've known all along, but didn't have the courage to be. The proof is in the low-fat pudding.

Lisa Pemberton

The Bargain

Do not wait for ideal circumstances, nor the best opportunities; they will never come.

Janet E. Stuart

I've always liked a bargain, so when my doctor sent me to a nutritionist after telling me that losing just five pounds of my excess weight could take thirty pounds of pressure off my aching knees, a deal was struck. I could easily lose a measly five pounds—I was sure of it.

The nutritionist, Nicole, laughed with me when I explained the bargain as she picked up my hand and seriously informed me that it was my best nutritional measure. Using my hand to illustrate proper portion sizes, my palm became the meat portion, my thumb, the fat portion, my fist the cooked vegetables (or fruit) and two fists for raw vegetables or salad.

I was shocked to realize that one can eat too much of a good thing, and that I'd been consuming vegetables sufficient for four or more people! Testing had revealed allergies to several grains, so I eliminated them for a time, later adding grains up to the size of my palm. It was very easy now to "eyeball" the right amount of food, even when we ate out. I would immediately push aside anything over that amount and save it for the "doggie bag" and the next day's portions. Then came the "E" word.

I love exercise—when I'm done. But starting is difficult, so in keeping with the five-pound bargain theme, motion was added to my day—five minutes at a time.

First, and most difficult, was the morning—five minutes of stretching. Rather than fight the urge to stay abed, I did several stretches IN bed! Stretching out one leg at a time, pressing each heel toward the end of the bed and holding for several seconds felt great, and I was comfortable repeating each side five times. Then raising each leg toward the ceiling, clasping my hands around the thigh, I pulled it toward me while holding a few seconds, again repeating each side five times, took half the five minutes. This wasn't as hard as I thought!

Second was choosing to park the car in the farthest spot from the building in the lot, forcing a five-minute walk to and from my vehicle. Still energized in the morning from the stay-in-bed "exercise," I practically crowed on the way in, and the walk out in the evening gave me a bit of time to review the upcoming evening or to plan dinner. Two of the three more times of motion were easily slipped into the workday—by climbing stairs the first five minutes of morning break and walking five minutes before lunch. The last segment of motion was saved for presleep stretching, or if I knew I had a long evening of appointments, I would increase both break and lunch segments by a few minutes and not worry about the evening.

Either way, I'd managed to painlessly add motion to every day! All this energy from five minutes here and there—what a bargain!

The last trick to the bargain was increasing water consumption. I'd playfully dubbed a friend the "water buffalo" for constantly carrying a half-gallon container of water, hiding secret thoughts of shame that I probably should, but never could, do that. My mistake, Nicole told me, was inviting failure by attempting to jump from barely finishing one to two eight-ounce glasses a day to eight full glasses. Instead, we planned for—yep, you guessed it— five smaller glasses. On arising, I chose warm water with a teaspoon of lemon juice, then another small glass of cold water before lunch and dinner, and one small glass of water or cup of tea with lunch and dinner. The juice-glass size relieved guilty feelings of defeat I got when I couldn't consume the entire contents of a large glass of water, and if I was still thirsty, having a second small glass became another tiny victory.

My goal for the bargain had been to lose one pound a week for five weeks, but that first week I lost the entire five pounds! I paid myself, putting the money I would have paid a weight management program for the week into a jar, and I planned to continue to pay myself weekly until I'd lost the other twenty pounds and had a fair amount of cash to purchase some new (smaller!) clothes. Perhaps the thought of smaller or better-fitting clothes is what motivated me to "up the ante" in consecutive weeks, as I knew it was unrealistic to expect that initial five-pound loss to repeat every week.

Breaking boredom was easy—but it was not without risk. Slipping a few minutes of exercise in as I waited in the copy room for the prints to roll out did gather a few smirks, raised eyebrows and outright laughter on occasion when someone unexpectedly entered the room while I was doing a squat or performing inhaling and exhaling Oxycise breathing exercises, which startled coworkers thought resembled Lamaze breathing for giving birth!

Bargaining is fun no matter what area of life I apply it to. It may have been mind over matter that made the difference as I battled and bargained five pounds at a time rather than holding up the entire goal, but I love bargains, and who wouldn't rather have five bargains for the "price" of one—no special equipment required!

Delores Christian Liesner

Stroke of Inspiration

Make your own recovery the first priority in your life.

Robin Norwood

It was one of those surreal moments. I was experiencing what was happening, but I was also outside myself, watching it. One minute I was standing at my desk dialing my phone. The next, I was looking at my right arm hanging limply by my side. My brain was telling me to raise my arm and continue dialing. My arm wasn't getting the message. In an instant, I knew I was having a stroke.

The ride to the ER seemed like a dream. My right arm wouldn't move, but I kept trying to force it to. My brain was spinning. Two things were certain—my arm wasn't working, and my obesity was the cause.

At age forty and weighing nearly 300 pounds, I ran a mental check of the past ten years. I had lost 127 pounds a few years before that, and I had successfully kept the weight off for almost six years. But for a number of reasons (or rather, excuses) I had managed to not only put the 127 pounds back on but an additional thirty. My mind went to all the times that I bypassed the exercise classes in favor of watching TV, all the times I had eaten pizza, fries, ice cream—anything but the healthy choices that had led to my weight-loss and maintenance success years earlier. I laid there in the ambulance and later in the hospital mourning the abilities that I had lost in a moment of time. And I laid there cursing myself for losing them due to my own poor choices.

Several grueling tests later, the cause of the stroke was found—an interaction of prescription medicines I was taking. I looked at the doctors in disbelief. My heart was healthy. My arteries were wide open. And the only thing wrong with my brain was the area damaged by the stroke. My weight and sedentary lifestyle didn't cause the stroke this time.

No matter the cause, I was still in a bad situation: my right hand not working, my balance gone, my nerves shattered. But I had a second chance to ensure that I would not have a stroke due to my lifestyle. And I seized it.

I immediately made plans. My mind was working overtime. I had used an exchange program the last time I had lost the weight. I knew that that was how I wanted to approach my eating again this time. The fried, sugary, buttery choices were gone from my view. Instead, the food pyramid was front and center.

But changing my eating habits was only part of the equation. I had to move again. I wanted to move again. And I prayed I would be able to. I thought back to the exercise classes I had taken. I watched the aerobics videos that I used to do. Heck—I watched the exercise video I was in! I knew I couldn't move like that right away, but I was determined to get to that point again. I laughed and cried. And I dug my heels in to fight the fight.

Exercise began as physical therapy for several months poststroke. Still, I sweat—literally and figuratively—

through three supervised sessions each week. And I "exercised" at home.

I worked hard to regain my balance and to regain the use of my hand. I kept the vision of myself doing an exercise video and walking around the neighborhood firmly in my site. I would watch *Sweatin' to the Oldies 3* and see myself moving like I used to. I thought of the time in the years before my stroke when I could have done those things and more, but I chose not to. That knowledge hurt.

I made slow changes to my eating. While I made much healthier choices, I was still eating too much. Too much of a good thing isn't much better than eating the "bad" things I had chosen in the past. The fact that I have always been an emotional eater didn't help in this situation.

Even though I had lost my ability to move quickly, my emotions didn't. I was on an hourly roller coaster, going from elation at the progress I was making to anger and regret to sadness and apathy, and ultimately, to fear.

Fear that I wouldn't recover the way I so desperately wanted to, fear that I would have another stroke, fear that I would die weighing 300 pounds. Fear that I would spend the rest of my life observing rather than participating. And as always, the emotions led me to reach for food. The difference was that instead of reaching for a candy bar, I was reaching for an apple or cereal.

It became obvious to me that what I was lacking was accountability in my eating. I was accountable in my exercise—the physical therapist saw to that by measuring and recording my progress several times a week. I needed the same for my eating program. So I joined Weight Watchers.

That was the absolute turning point in the path to my full recovery. I got the point, so to speak. I am now counting what I am eating and relearning portion control. Weighing in weekly makes me accountable for the choices

I make during the week. It helps keep me honest with myself. Journaling is the key for me. If I don't write down what I've eaten, I "forget" about the fact that I have used up those points for the day. It has to be in black and white and, thankfully, in my own handwriting. My food journal is tangible evidence of what I'm doing right—and what I'm doing wrong.

I'm a people person. I always have been. But my stroke made me more introspective and reserved. That is another area in which Weight Watchers has proven to be a huge benefit.

The camaraderie of the weekly meetings is not only inspiring, it is fun. We cheer each other on, and I look forward to seeing the people who have come to be my Sunday afternoon friends. It is much more fun to share this journey than to walk the road alone. And it is much harder to give up when you know there is a group of people looking forward to seeing you each week.

Exercise is still a challenge for me. My balance isn't 100 percent and never will be. But I can't and won't let that stop me. I can't imagine choosing not to move after not being able to. I've always heard that you don't know what you've got 'til it's gone . . . but I never truly understood the truth in those words.

By the grace of God, with a lot of help from others and buckets of my own sweat and tears, I can do *Sweatin' 3* again, and I can walk confidently around the neighborhood. There are still many evenings when I don't feel like exercising, but I do anyway. I do because I can—and that's a wonderful gift to make the most of.

I carry reminders of my "stroke of inspiration" every day. Most people would not notice them, but I do and I'm grateful for them. They are reminders of how far I've come and of where I don't want to find myself again. I am on the path to total health, and it's a fun and exciting road to take again.

I have lost over fifty pounds at this point. I have a long way to go . . . but I've come a long, long way already. Life is good.

Charmi Schroeder

Couch Meets Table

Do not dwell in the past, do not dream of the future; concentrate the mind on the present moment.

Buddha

You're probably familiar with the expression "You are what you eat." For me, it was more like: "You are WHERE you eat." Either way, the result wasn't pretty.

My postage stamp-sized kitchen precluded a table or even an eating bar, and the dining room table was covered with books, magazines and files, not to mention two cats basking in the sun from the only south-facing window. Even if I could have cleared a spot on the table, one of my favorite cooking shows aired at suppertime and the TV sat in the living room.

So I ended up eating on the couch.

Although an avid fan of the Food Channel, I spent so much time watching TV I didn't have time to try out the recipes and techniques. I did most of what passed for cooking during commercials. When you only had two minutes to whip up something remotely edible, you

quickly learned to ignore words like flambé, sauté and juli-
enne and substitute microwave or delivery.

My motto was: If it couldn't be nuked or delivered, I
didn't eat it.

Eating on the couch led to several problems. It was
impossible to watch TV, balance a plate on my lap and cut
food all at the same time without dropping half the contents on the cushions. Although my cats liked the arrange-
ment and vied for who got to sit next to me while I ate, I
was less happy. To cut down on cleaning bills, I gravitated
toward finger foods. Pizza, chicken nuggets, chips and
cookies were a lot easier to manage than linguini with
tomatoes concasse or osso buco.

The combination of food and TV meant I often finished
an entire meal without any recollection of having eaten it.
Bags of chips and cookies disappeared the same way.

The other day when I struggled yet again to zip up my
favorite pants, I discovered a more immediate problem.
Eating dinner while watching food shows had not only
expanded my culinary vocabulary, it had also broadened
my beam.

It was time to take action. For my first step, I turned off
the TV. Since I couldn't enlarge my kitchen, I rolled up my
sleeves and cleared off the dining room table. While the
cats were not too happy about losing their favorite spots,
the dining room looked much more inviting without
mounds of papers cluttering up every surface.

Next, I opened a cookbook and started to plan healthy
meals. I visited my local grocery store and took a shopping
cart for a ride through the produce aisles and the meat and
fish departments—hitherto strange and forbidding terri-
tory. Then I introduced myself to mixing bowls, pots and
pans, and a large appliance in my kitchen called a stove.

Cooking proved more difficult than I had thought. What
looks simple on TV seldom turns out that way in real life.

I had neither a sous chef nor a clean-up crew to help out.

I made many discoveries on my culinary journey. One, when the recipe says one cup, it means one cup, not half a cup or two cups. Two, substituting ingredients can be a recipe for disaster. And three, four-year-old spices don't have much flavor left in them. Many a dish I prepared went straight from oven to garbage can.

Along the way, I also learned that simple was best. That flambé means you'd better have the fire department on speed dial. And that if a recipe calls for ingredients you can't pronounce, turn the page and try one you can actually say.

To be honest, I backslid a few times when my traitorous fingers dialed for pizza. But I persevered.

I started to enjoy cooking. I played around with textures and ate more raw or lightly grilled vegetables instead of relying on that old standby—the potato. I started using herbs and spices instead of salt, fat and sugar to flavor food. I bought a couple of new cookbooks that emphasized healthy cooking and continued experimenting with different recipes.

As a surprising side effect, now that I could actually taste my food, I found myself eating less and enjoying it more. And since I felt funny eating chips or a chocolate bar at the dining room table, which was the only place I now ate, I gradually stopped buying them. Within a couple of months, I lost fifteen pounds without dieting and without feeling deprived or hungry.

As for my favorite cooking show? I tape it and watch it later—after I've eaten.

Harriet Cooper

Worship Walk

You will praise the name of the LORD your God,
who has worked wonders for you.

Joel 2:26 NIV

It's been two years, and I can't believe that I've stayed on my low-carb diet. I say "low-carb" because I know that my body needs some carbs. Otherwise, I'd fall off my treadmill. That's another thing that amazes me—that I've stuck with my motorized treadmill. It's just not like me to stick to something hard without losing my way. No sugar. No honey. And no molasses. None of my favorite foods— like Krispy Kreme doughnuts, brownies, fluffy biscuits and sweet corn bread—are on my diet. I miss them nearly every day. Every muffin I bake is from scratch, and not quite the same with Splenda and soy flour, but it's livable, and I have lost over forty pounds.

As a diabetic, not only is my glucose level under control, but my hemoglobin levels have dropped from a poor reading of 7.5 down to a nearly normal 6.3. The lower my score is, the less likely I am to lose a foot or kidney function or my life! So my diet is not only life-changing, but it is life saving. And frankly, I could not have done this without the grace of God. I just don't have that kind of willpower. That is why I call every day, on or off of my treadmill, eating only foods that are good for my body, my worship walk.

My goal is simple. I am never ahead of my present meal or snack. This is a walk that I take moment by moment, always remembering what doughnuts taste like. If I plan ahead, or if I look toward tomorrow, I know that I'll fail.

There are two pictures of me that I like to compare. One is of me holding my birthday balloons, two years ago. I'm laughing at my family, and you can tell that I have a happy life. The other picture is more recent. It's of me sitting on my husband's lap, as we smile into the camera. The difference in me is not only that I'm slimmer, but that I can actually fit on my husband's lap! For me, that says everything.

This has not been easy. I am not a woman who heads for the dieting magazine. I'm the one who's drooling over the chocolate cake. Strangely enough, I still bake for my family. In fact, I do more baking for them since I know I'm not going to eat it. I do, however, get to take that first sniff, if there is a bag of doughnuts around. "Wait! Don't open it! Let me!" Mmmmmhhh! What a wonderful smell! Then I move on to my high-protein blueberry muffin and thank God there is such a thing as toasted soy flour and Splenda.

When I met my husband, I was 120 pounds. On the outside I looked confidant, but inside I was a mess. I believed that if I lost my youth and my perfect figure, my husband could not love me. Why? Because I did not love myself. Now, at sixty, I realize that my view of myself and of my husband's love was shallow. My husband and I will soon be married for twenty-five years. During our marriage, he has told me every day how beautiful I am to him. His love, support and faithfulness have been constant, yet only now do I believe him. Only now, at sixty, and a mere 160 pounds, do I believe that I'm beautiful.

There are diet books enough, and the Internet is full of diets, but it was not the diet that was my problem. It was the reflection that I saw of myself, not in the mirror, but in my heart. So today is a good day. It's a day that begins anew, in a walk that is both physical and spiritual, a worship walk that I can only take from moment to moment, as I place my hand in the hand of God.

Jaye Lewis

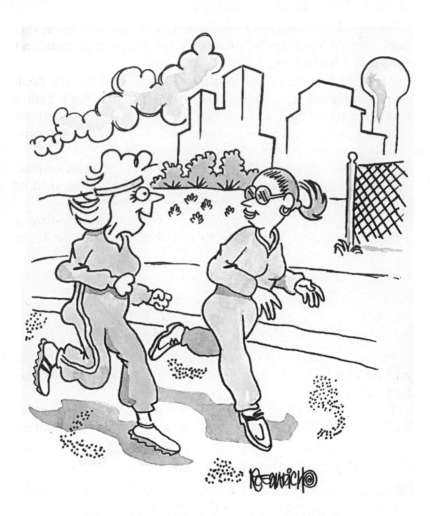

"One thing I like about my new image
is that there's so much less of it!"

Reprinted by permission of Dan Rosanditch.

More Chicken Soup?

We would love to hear your reactions to the stories in this book. Please let us know what your favorite stories were and how they affected you.

Many of the stories and poems you have read in this book were submitted by readers like you who had read earlier *Chicken Soup for the Soul* books. We publish at least five or six *Chicken Soup for the Soul* books every year. We invite you to contribute a story to one of these future volumes.

Stories may be up to 1,200 words and must uplift or inspire. You may submit an original piece, something you have read or your favorite quotation on your refrigerator door.

To obtain a copy of our submission guidelines and a listing of upcoming *Chicken Soup* books, please write, fax or check our websites. Please send your submissions to:

Chicken Soup for the Soul
P.O. Box 30880 • Santa Barbara, CA 93130
fax: 805-563-2945
website: www. chickensoup.com

Just send a copy of your stories and other pieces to the above address. We will be sure that both you and the author are credited for your submission.

For information about speaking engagements, other books, audiotapes, workshops and training programs, please contact any of our authors directly.

The Optimal Weight for Life (OWL) Program

The publisher and authors of *Chicken Soup for the Dieter's Soul* are pleased to donate five cents for every book sold to the Optimal Weight for Life Program at Children's Hospital, Boston.

OWL is a multidisciplinary care clinic dedicated to the evaluation and treatment of children who are overweight/obese.

As the largest hospital-based pediatric obesity program in New England, OWL provides more than 500 new patients each year with state-of-the-art care. OWL features innovative treatments for pediatric obesity developed through clinical research and promotes public awareness and prevention efforts.

At OWL specialists in nutrition, endocrinology, developmental pediatrics and behavioral medicine develop successful lifestyle interventions for obese children and adolescents.

New patients are evaluated to identify any underlying medical conditions (such as a hormone problem) and potential complications (including high cholesterol, diabetes or gastrointestinal disease).

Patients are given nutritional counseling and families meet privately with a dietitian to discuss practical aspects of starting the recommended individualized meal plan.

OWL provides a combination of short-term individual and family psychotherapy sessions to increase motivation to change diet and physical activity levels. These treatments may also help children cope with the emotional stresses associated with being overweight.

Group therapy is offered on a periodic basis to facilitate individual treatment. Groups generally meet for ninety minutes each week for a total of six weeks. Participation by the child and at least one parent/guardian is required. For more information contact:

www.childrenshospital.org/OWL
Optimal Weight for Life Program
Children's Hospital, Boston
300 Longwood Avenue • Boston, MA 02115
phone: (617) 355-5159 • fax: (617) 730-0505

Who Is Jack Canfield?

Jack Canfield is the cocreator and editor of the Chicken Soup for the Soul series, which *Time* magazine has called "the publishing phenomenon of the decade." The series now has 105 titles with over 100 million copies in print in forty-one languages. Jack is also the coauthor of eight other bestselling books, including *The Success Principles: How to Get from Where You Are to Where You Want to Be, Dare to Win, The Aladdin Factor, You've Got to Read This Book,* and *The Power of Focus: How to Hit Your Business, Personal and Financial Targets with Absolute Certainty.*

Jack has recently developed a telephone coaching program and an online coaching program based on his most recent book, *The Success Principles.* He also offers a seven-day Breakthrough to Success seminar every summer, which attracts 400 people from fifteen countries around the world.

Jack is the CEO of Chicken Soup for the Soul Enterprises and the Canfield Training Group in Santa Barbara, California, and founder of the Foundation for Self-Esteem in Culver City, California. He has conducted intensive personal and professional development seminars on the principles of success for over 900,000 people in twenty-one countries around the world. He has spoken to hundreds of thousands of others at numerous conferences and conventions and has been seen by millions of viewers on national television shows such as *The Today Show, Fox and Friends, Inside Edition, Hard Copy,* CNN's *Talk Back Live, 20/20, Eye to Eye,* and the *NBC Nightly News* and the *CBS Evening News.*

Jack is the recipient of many awards and honors, including three honorary doctorates and a Guinness World Records Certificate for having seven Chicken Soup for the Soul books appearing on the *New York Times* bestseller list on May 24, 1998.

To write to Jack or for inquiries about Jack as a speaker, his coaching programs or his seminars, use the following contact information:

Jack Canfield
The Canfield Companies
P.O. Box 30880
Santa Barbara, CA 93130
Phone: 805-563-2935 • Fax: 805-563-2945
E-mail: info@jackcanfield.com
website: www.jackcanfield.com

Who Is Mark Victor Hansen?

In the area of human potential, no one is more respected than Mark Victor Hansen. For more than thirty years, Mark has focused solely on helping people from all walks of life reshape their personal vision of what's possible. His powerful messages of possibility, opportunity and action have created powerful change in thousands of organizations and millions of individuals worldwide.

He is a sought-after keynote speaker, bestselling author and marketing maven. Mark's credentials include a lifetime of entrepreneurial success and an extensive academic background. He is a prolific writer with many bestselling books, such as *The One Minute Millionaire, The Power of Focus, The Aladdin Factor* and *Dare to Win*, in addition to the *Chicken Soup for the Soul* series. Mark has made a profound influence through his library of audios, videos and articles in the areas of big thinking, sales achievement, wealth building, publishing success, and personal and professional development.

Mark is the founder of the MEGA Seminar Series. MEGA Book Marketing University and Building Your MEGA Speaking Empire are annual conferences where Mark coaches and teaches new and aspiring authors, speakers and experts on building lucrative publishing and speaking careers. Other MEGA events include MEGA Marketing Magic and My MEGA Life.

He has appeared on television (*Oprah*, CNN and *The Today Show*), in print (*Time, U.S. News & World Report, USA Today, New York Times* and *Entrepreneur*) and on countless radio interviews, assuring our planet's people that "you can easily create the life you deserve."

As a philanthropist and humanitarian, Mark works tirelessly for organizations such as Habitat for Humanity, American Red Cross, March of Dimes, Childhelp USA and many others. He is the recipient of numerous awards that honor his entrepreneurial spirit, philanthropic heart and business acumen. He is a lifetime member of the Horatio Alger Association of Distinguished Americans, an organization that honored Mark with the prestigious Horatio Alger Award for his extraordinary life achievements.

Mark Victor Hansen is an enthusiastic crusader of what's possible and is driven to make the world a better place.

Mark Victor Hansen & Associates, Inc.
P.O. Box 7665
Newport Beach, CA 92658
Phone: 949-764-2640 • Fax: 949-722-6912
Website: www.markvictorhansen.com

Who Is Theresa Peluso?

Theresa has always felt drawn to a page and the power of words. Books represent knowledge, expression, freedom, adventure, creativity and escape—so it's no surprise that her career has revolved around books.

Theresa's career began over thirty years ago in a large publisher's book club operation. In 1981, Theresa joined Health Communications, a fledgling book publisher that grew to become the country's #1 self-help publisher and home to groundbreaking *New York Times* bestsellers and the series recognized as a publishing phenomenon, *Chicken Soup for the Soul*.

After twenty years spent in the day-to-day operations of a thriving publishing company, Theresa is now developing books as a writer, compiler and editor.

She is the coauthor of *Chicken Soup for the Horse Lover's Soul, Chicken Soup for the Horse Lover's Soul II, Chicken Soup for the Recovering Soul,* its companion *Chicken Soup for the Recovering Soul Daily Inspirations* and *Chicken Soup for the Shopper's Soul.*

In addition to other *Chicken Soup* books waiting to be hatched, Theresa is developing titles in the *Read a Little Bit About . . .* series. *Read a Little Bit* books help teens and young adults build literacy skills while focusing on relevant, contemporary topics and issues, such as buying a car or getting a job. Theresa is also working on *Sonic Boomers: That Sound You Hear Is YOU Making a Difference,* a book featuring unsung heroes of the baby boomer generation who have found fulfillment and growth in their lives by helping others.

Theresa lives in South Florida with her husband Brian and two cats who think they are dogs. All of her diligence and good dieting flies out the window at the first sign of a hurricane when her need for comfort food (Cheez Doodles and chocolate—not at the same time) kicks into high gear. You can contact Theresa at:

teri@dieterssoul.com
Health Communications, Inc.
3201 SW 15th Street • Deerfield Beach, FL 33442
phone: 954-360-0909 • fax: 954-418-0844

Contributors

The stories in this book are original pieces or taken from previously published sources, such as books, magazines and newspapers. If you would like to contact any of the contributors for information about their writing or would like to invite them to speak in your community, look for their contact information included in their biography.

Kate Baggott is a Canadian writer living in Europe. Her essays, articles and short stories have appeared in the *Globe and Mail*, the *Christian Science Monitor* and *Technology Review* among other publications. Links to recent pieces can be found at www.katebaggott.com.

Suzanne Baginskie recently retired from her job as a law office manager/paralegal for more than twenty-five years. She has been published in other *Chicken Soup for the Soul* books, *Cat's Magazine, True Romance* and has written several nonfiction articles. She lives on the west coast of Florida with her husband, Al.

Karen A. Bakhazi is a new writer who enjoys coffee trips and working with the girls in her church's youth group where she is inspired by watching the kids learn and grow spiritually. She and her husband enjoy frequent trips to Disneyland where you never have to grow up!

Jessica Blaire lives in Michigan and currently works as a travel editor for a webzine. From yoga to rock climbing to chasing her hyperactive four-legged furry roommate down the street, she fits exercise into her daily schedule and lives for the delicious concoctions found at her local natural grocery store.

Guy Burdick is a Washington, D.C.-based editor and writer who has type 2 diabetes. He lives in Alexandria, Virginia, with this wife, Suzanne Kelly, and their adopted shelter pets. He currently is working on a book about his experiences, *Difficult Run: From Diabetic Coma to the Marine Corps Marathon*.

Kathe M. Campbell lives on a western Montana mountain with her precious keeshond and a few kitties where she raises champion mammoth donkeys. Three grown children, eleven grandkids and three great-grandchildren round out the herd. Her Montana stories are found on many e-zines. Kathe is a contributing author to the *Chicken Soup for the Soul* series, *People Who Make a Difference*, and various anthologies, magazines and medical journals.

Sally Clark lives in Fredericksburg, Texas, and still shops incognito at the same grocery store. Her humor work has appeared in *America's Funniest Humor! Book Two* and *GreenPrints: The Weeder's Digest*. Sally also writes and publishes award-winning poetry, nonfiction, children's stories and greeting cards. Contact her at auslande@ktc.com.

Harriet Cooper is a writer living in Toronto, Canada. She specializes in humorous and serious articles and essays on diet, health, the environment, family, relationships and cats. She also writes short stories and humorous verse. Her work has appeared in numerous national and international magazines, e-zines, websites, newspapers and anthologies.

Barbara A. Croce is now a certified personal trainer, working on location and out of her home. She attributes her success to Jesus, her Lord. She lives with her best friend and husband of twenty-six years, Rich. You can check out both her websites at www.glorywriter.4t.com and www.barbsfitu.com.

Suzan Davis is the author of *Babes on Blades: Drop Physical, Mental and Spiritual Flab Through Inline Skating* and is a frequent *Chicken Soup for the Soul* contributor. Suzan's public relations firm promotes exercise and healthy living. She lives in California with two charming children and two naughty dogs. Suzan swears life begins after forty. Contact her at suzandavis@sbcglobal.net.

Marilyn Eudaly lives in Texas with her husband and faithful dog, Hairy Truman. Her daughter, who is mentioned here, lives nearby and is her writing mentor. Marilyn is a member of Romance Writers of America, American Christian Fiction Writers and the North Texas Romance Writers of America.

Greg Faherty has had several fiction and nonfiction stories and poems published, including one in *Chicken Soup for the Teenage Soul IV*. When he and his wife are not exercising with their dogs or cooking healthy meals, he owns and operates www.a-perfect-resume.com, and also provides proofreading and editing services.

Susan Farr-Fahncke is dedicated to making a difference. Susan is the creator of www.2theheart.com, the founder of the volunteer group, Angels2TheHeart, and a busy author. With stories featured in several *Chicken Soup for the Soul* books, she is also the author of the beloved *Angel's Legacy*. Susan teaches online writing workshops, and you can sign up for a workshop and see more of her writing at www.2theheart.com.

Tricia Finch is a former youth librarian, now a stay-at-home mom and free-lance writer. She lives in Venice, Florida, with her husband Jeff, son Nicholas, two dogs and two cats. She enjoys reading, scrapbooking and having fun with her family. Tricia's credits include *Venice Gulf Coast Living, Southwest Florida Parent and Child,* and book reviews for *School Library Journal* and *KLIATT*.

Jacquelyn B. Fletcher is a full-time freelance writer who has written hundreds of magazine articles in addition to nonfiction books, young adult fiction, brochures, Web content and a variety of other projects in the name of her motto: Will Write for Food. Contact her at jacquebfletcher@aol.com.

Peggy Frezon is a freelance writer from upstate New York. She is a frequent contributor to *Guideposts, Sweet 16, Positive Thinking* and *Angels on Earth,* and her work has appeared in *Teaching Tolerance* and *Chicken Soup for the Kid's Soul 2*. She enjoys playing with her dogs, Hudson and Kelly. You can e-mail Peggy at ecritMeg@nycap.rr.com.

James Hammill is a business analyst with ANALYTIC*i* in New York. He lives in Caldwell, New Jersey, with wife Astrida and has two sons, Chris and Greg. James loves singing bass with the locally popular a capella group Wide Variety. You can e-mail James from the group's Web site, www.widevariety.com.

Julia Havey is eDiets' "Master Motivator" and a bestselling author. She lost 130 pounds, and she proves that healthy eating and motivation can change a person's life—not through deprivation but through the realization of belief in one's own abilities to succeed. Julia's book, *The Vice Busting Diet,* is endorsed by Dr. David L. Katz, M.D., Dr. Mehmet Oz and the amazing Mark Victor Hansen. Visit her website at: www.ViceBustingDiet.com.

Jonny Hawkins is a full-time cartoonist from Sherwood, Michigan. Thousands of his cartoons have been published in magazines, books and other publications over the last twenty-one years. His annual calendars, *Medical Cartoon-A-Day* and *Fishing Cartoon-A-Day* are available everywhere. He can be reached at jonnyhawkins2nz@yahoo.com.

Selena Hayes is a freelance writer at heart and a secretary by demand. The proud Canuck lives in beautiful British Columbia, Canada, with her husband and three children. Her advice for successful weight loss—cut your hair, dress lightly and wear smaller jewelry. It's all about having fun!

Lori Hein (LoriHein.com) is the author of *Ribbons of Highway: A Mother-Child Journey Across America* and a contributor to *Chicken Soup for the Horse Lover's Soul II.* Lori's writing has appeared in publications nationwide and online. She publishes a world travel blog at www.ribbonsofhighway.blogspot.com.

Jan Henrikson savors the occasional bite of chocolate in Tucson, Arizona. She is the editor of *Eat by Choice, Not by Habit,* by Sylvia Haskvitz (Puddle Dancer Press, 2005) and managing editor of Dr. Becky Coleman's newsletter, *The Wave* (www.o-c-e-a-n.com). You can reach her at jan@o-c-e-a-n.com.

Samantha Hoffman wrote her first short story in third grade. Her work can be found in *The Corner Magazine* in London, *The Sidewalk's End* and *LongStoryShort.* She lives and writes in Chicago, where she's working on her novel. Samantha can be contacted at samanthahoffman@aol.com.

Georgia A. Hubley retired after twenty years in financial management to write her memoirs. She's a frequent contributor to the *Chicken Soup for the Soul* series and numerous national magazines and newspapers. She has two grown sons and resides with her husband in Henderson, Nevada. You can reach Georgia at GEOHUB@aol.com.

Jennie Ivey lives in Cookeville, Tennessee. She is a newspaper columnist and author of two books, *Tennessee Tales the Textbooks Don't Tell* and *E Is For Elvis.* She has published numerous fiction and nonfiction pieces, including stories in three *Chicken Soup for the Soul* anthologies: *Horse Lover's Soul, Life Lessons for Women,* and *Healthy Living: Menopause.* Contact her at jivey@frontiernet.net.

Janet Marianne Jackson is a passionate writer and traveler; most of her published articles are based on her traveling experiences. Janet is also keenly interested in health and fitness matters and as a former scientist still keeps a hand in medical and technical writing.

Roberta Beach Jacobson has twenty-six cats and two dogs. She writes for *True Confessions, Playgirl* and *True Experience*. Visit www.travelwriters.com/Roberta.

Edwina L. Kaikai is an award-winning journalist and author of *Stomach in My Lap*, a frank, motivating chronicle of her fitness journey. She's passionate about staying fit and helping others get there, too, via her example, book, website and speaking engagements. She's just a click away at www.emptylap.com.

Colleen Kappeler is a freelance writer, editor and writing teacher. Colleen has written personal essays for several national magazines and has worked with hundreds of writers over the past seven years. She works with writers to help them discover and invest in their writing passion. Visit www.wisconsinwriters.com.

Susan A. Karas owns and operates a business with her husband. In her free time she shops and enjoys visiting with her two grown children, who just moved out into their own places. Susan is a regular contributor to *Guideposts Magazine* and has been published in *Sweet 16, PLUS Magazine* and *Guideposts 4 Kids*. She can be reached at Mssusankaras@yahoo.com.

Candy Killion has contributed to *Chicken Soup for the Soul Healthy Living: Menopause* and *Chicken Soup for the Recovering Soul: Daily Inspirations*. She lives near Fort Lauderdale, Florida, with her husband John and—of course—Max.

Jerry King is a prolific, versatile cartoonist and the author and illustrator of seven nationally published cartoon books. He has also illustrated ten children's books and has provided illustrations for numerous children's publications. One of Jerry's cartoon characters has been made into a stuffed animal. See more of his work at www.jerryking.com.

Deborah P. Kolodji is a native Southern Californian who works in information technology to support her book-buying habits and to pay for her children's ever-increasing college tuition. Her story, "A River Runs Through Me," appeared in the anthology, *Charity*, by Red Rock Press, and she has published hundreds of poems in journals both on and off the Web.

Nancy Julien Kopp has published stories, articles, essays, children's stories and poetry in magazines, newspapers, online and in anthologies including *Chicken Soup for the Father and Daughter Soul* and *Chicken Soup for the Sister's Soul II*. Nancy is a former teacher who still enjoys teaching via the written word.

Jaye Lewis is an award-winning writer who, at age sixty, finds that the trials of life and its lessons are the best way to find out who she is. You can read more of Jaye's inspirational stories on her website at www.entertainingangels.org or e-mail Jaye at jayelewis@comcast.net.

Delores Christian Liesner lives life passionately and humorously, revealing dynamic hope and confidence found in the Heavenly Heritage of our personal God. She writes from Racine, Wisconsin. Best jewels are husband Ken, children and grandchildren. Delores is a CLASS graduate. E-mail Delores at delores7faith@yahoo.com.

Terry A. Lilley is a long-time resident of New Mexico, where foods are full of flavor and every meal is an invitation to a celebration. In between the fiestas, she takes time for the siesta and the occasional bit of passionate gardening.

Gary Luerding resides in southern Oregon with Lynne, his wife of forty-four years. He is a frequent *Chicken Soup* contributor with "Beyond the Breakers" (*Fisherman's Soul*), "The Honeymoon is Over" (*Military Wife's Soul*), "My Mother's Piano" (*Mother's and Son's Soul*) and "The Sunny Side" (*Cup of Comfort for Mothers and Sons*) and author of *Inshore Ocean Fishing for Dummies*.

Michelle May, M.D. is the award-winning author of *Am I Hungry? What to Do When Diets Don't Work*. She founded the Am I Hungry?® Weight Management Program, dedicated to changing the way people think about eating and exercise. You'll find book excerpts, workshops, resources and presentations for your organization at www.AmIHungry.com.

Michelle McLean is twenty-nine-year-old mother of two. She has a BS in history, will soon begin work on her master's and is an avid writer. Michelle does some freelance work and is currently working on getting some children's stories and her first novel published.

Ann Morrow and her family live in Custer, South Dakota, where she writes humor/inspirational pieces. Her columns and short stories have appeared in various publications, including previous *Chicken Soup for the Soul* books. Please write to Ann at nova@gwtc.net.

Mark Parisi's "off the mark" comic panel has been syndicated since 1987 and is distributed by United Media. Mark's humor also graces greeting cards, T-shirts, calendars, magazines, newsletters and books. Please visit his website at www.offthemark.com. Lynn is his wife/business partner, and their daughter, Jenny, contributes with inspiration (as do three cats).

Lisa Pemberton resides in Hannibal, Missouri. She shares her life with husband, Brad, her children, Brandon and Lyndsay, and extended family and close friends. Her company provides professional services to speakers and meeting planners. Hobbies include writing, coaching and genealogy. Contact Lisa at www.professionalspeakerservices.com or psslisa@wdemail.com.

Ava Pennington is a writer, Bible study teacher, public speaker and former human resources director. With an MBA from St. John's University in New York, and a Bible Studies certificate from Moody Bible Institute in Chicago, Ava divides her time between teaching, writing, speaking and volunteering. Contact her at rusavapen@yahoo.com.

Perry P. Perkins is a Christian novelist born and raised in Oregon. His writing includes *Just Past Oysterville* and *Shoalwater Voices*. Perry is a student of Jerry B. Jenkins Christian Writer's Guild and a frequent contributor to the *Chicken Soup for the Soul* anthologies. Enjoy Perry's work at www.perryperkinsbooks.com.

Pamela Wertz Peterson is a native of the Midwest who now lives in Santa Cruz, California, with husband, Mike, and tortoiseshell cat, Jazz. Passions include dream work, women's spirituality, gardening, reading, cooking and travel. Pamela's career path has veered from special education teacher to cooking school owner to private tutor to writer.

Stephanie Piro lives in New Hampshire with her husband, daughter and three cats. She is one of King Features' team of women cartoonists, the "Six Chix" (she is the Saturday chick!). Her single panel, "Fair Game," appears in newspapers and on her website: www.stephaniepiro.com. She also designs gift items for her company Strip T's. Contact her at stephaniepiro@verizon.net or 27 River Road, Farmington, NH, 03835.

Felice Prager is a freelance writer from Scottsdale, Arizona, with credits in local, national and international publications. In addition to writing, she also works with adults and children with moderate to severe learning disabilities as a multisensory educational therapist.

Dan Rosandich owns and operates www.danscartoons.com, which is an extensive online database featuring three thousand of Dan's best cartoons. The images are archived by subject matter to easily locate specific cartoons. Dan also specializes in creating custom cartoons and has been extensively published in most major magazines. E-mail dan@danscartoons.com with questions.

Linda Sago lives in Billings, Montana, with six cats and a large dog who is sure he is a cat! A freelance writer, she has written for *Fit Magazine* and *Guideposts*. Check out her story, two cookbooks, before/after pictures and weight-loss kit found at www.cu.imt.net/~gedison/emerald.

Charmi Schroeder is a freelance writer and speaker. She has appeared on several national television shows and in *Sweatin' to the Oldies 3* and has owned her own motivational speaking and fitness business, appropriately named No Limits. She currently works as a systems analyst while pursuing her passion for writing.

Laura Schroll is a freelance writer living on Long Island, New York. Her essays and articles have appeared in various publications including *Tea, A MAGAZINE, ByLine, The Detroit Free Press* and *A Cup of Comfort for Mothers to Be*.

Ken Shane is a songwriter from New Jersey. He is also the music columnist for the monthly newsmagazine *NYC Plus* and a frequent contributor to *The Aquarian Weekly*. He is currently collaborating on a novel based on the songs from his first album. Visit him at www.kenshane.com.

Deborah H. Shouse is a speaker, writer and editor. Her writing has appeared in *Reader's Digest, Newsweek* and *Spirituality & Health*. She is donating all proceeds from her book, *Love in the Land of Dementia: Finding Hope in the Caregiver's Journey*, to Alzheimer's programs and research. Please visit Deborah on the Web at www.thecreativityconnection.com.

Jean Stewart is an editor and writer in Mission Viejo, California, whose stories can be found in *Chicken Soup for the Father & Daughter Soul* and *Horse Lover's Soul II*, as well as *Cup of Comfort for Women in Love*. She also writes travel and parenting articles and is working on books for mothers and grandmothers, since she and her husband dote on their twin daughters and two grandchildren.

Ken Swarner is author of *Whose Kids Are These Anyway?* (Penquin/Putnam). He can be reached at kenswarner@aol.com.

Sandra L. Tatara has had several short stories published, including a story in the 2003 edition of *Chicken Soup for the Horse Lover's Soul*. She raises registered quarter horses, paints in several mediums and is a hospice volunteer. She now has two grandchildren, and her first novel, *Remember Me*, is scheduled for publication in May 2007.

B. J. Taylor battles the temptations of the fridge and the cupboards daily. She is an award-winning author whose work has appeared in *Guideposts*, many Chicken Soup books, and numerous magazines and newspapers. She has a wonderful husband, four children and two adorable grandsons. You can reach B. J. through her website at www.clik.to/bjtaylor.

Ed VanDeMark is a career public servant, freelance writer and cartoonist. He and wife, Linda, have three adult children and five grandchildren. His interests include church, reading, gardening, human temperament and baseball.

Aly Walansky is the managing editor of *HOOTERS Magazine* as well as a freelance editor and writer based in New York City. Her hobbies include shopping, martini lounges and rocking out to her favorite indie bands. Visit her website at www.mediabistro.com/alywalansky.

Debra Weaver is a writer and educator with experience across a wide range of audiences. She has taught students from preschool to high school and trained adults in workplace skills. Her books include *50 Ways to Eat Your Veggies* and *The Guerilla Guide to Free Online Classes*.

Permissions *(continued from page iv)*

Chocolate Is Not the Enemy. Reprinted by permission of Jan Henrikson. ©2005 Jan Henrikson.

A Can of Peas and a Jog Around the Block. Reprinted by permission of Lori Hein. ©2006 Lori Hein.

Take Two. Reprinted by permission of Karen A Bakhazi. ©2005 Karen A Bakhazi.

You Choose, You Lose. Reprinted by permission of B. J. Taylor. ©2006 B. J. Taylor.

Whatever I Want. Reprinted by permission of Perry P. Perkins. ©2006 Perry P. Perkins.

Finally Success—A New Me! Reprinted by permission of Sandra L. Tatara. ©2006 Sandra L. Tatara.

The Mirror Doesn't Lie. Reprinted by permission of Candy Killion. ©2006 Candy Killion.

The Thighs Have It. Reprinted by permission of Deborah H. Shouse. ©2006 Deborah H. Shouse.

Where Money Meets Resolutions. Reprinted by permission of Harriet Cooper. ©2005 Harriet Cooper.

No Pizza? No Problem! Reprinted by permission of Aly Walansky. ©2006 Aly Walansky.

Morning Walk. Reprinted by permission of Deborah P. Kolodji. ©2004 Deborah P. Kolodji.

Gone to the Dogs. Reprinted by permission of Greg Faherty. ©2006 Greg Faherty.

Skinny Munchies. Reprinted by permission of Sally Clark. ©2006 Sally Clark. Originally appeared on www.humorpress.com, Dec. 2005/Jan. 2006.

Trading Fat Cells for Barbells. Reprinted by permission of Suzan Davis. ©2001 Suzan Davis. Previously published in *Chicken Soup for the Soul Healthy Living, Weight Loss* (Health Communications, Inc., 2004), *Granite Bay View* (2002) and *Fitness and Speed Skating Times* (2002).

The Exchange Rate. Reprinted by permission of Harriet Cooper. ©2005 Harriet Cooper.

Facing the Lady in the Mirror. Reprinted by permission of Barbara A. Croce. ©2004 Barbara A. Croce.

A Diet for Life—Literally. Reprinted by permission of Jessica Blaire. ©2006 Jessica Blaire.

A Skinny By-Product. Reprinted by permission of Ed VanDeMark. ©2006 Ed VanDeMark.

My Own Way. Reprinted by permission of Colleen Kappeler. ©2006 Colleen Kappeler.

Weight-Loss Wisdom from a Toddler. Reprinted by permission of Tricia Finch. ©2006 Tricia Finch.

10 Tricks to Help You Stay on Your Diet. Reprinted by permission of Felice Prager. ©2003 Felice Prager.

Slow and Steady. Reprinted by permission of Ken Shane. ©2006 Ken Shane.

Thin! Nine Years . . . and Counting! Reprinted by permission of Linda Sago. ©2006 Linda Sago.

Peel-a-Pound Soup. Reprinted by permission of Gary Luerding. ©2004 Gary Luerding.

Running from a Diabetic Coma to the Marine Corps Marathon. Reprinted by permission of Guy Burdick. ©2006 Guy Burdick.

What's the Point? Reprinted by permission of Ken Swarner. ©2003 Ken Swarner. Previously published in *Chicken Soup for the Soul Healthy Living, Weight Loss* (Health Communications, Inc., 2004).

The Road to Self-Worth. Reprinted by permission of Jacquelyn B. Fletcher. ©2004 Jacquelyn B. Fletcher. Previously published in *Chicken Soup for the Soul Healthy Living, Weight Loss* (Health Communications, Inc., 2004).

Stop Dieting, Start Living. Reprinted by permission of Michelle May, M.D. ©2005 Michelle May, M.D. Portions excerpted from *Am I Hungry? What to Do When Diets Don't Work* (self-published).

One Newspaper at a Time. Reprinted by permission of Michelle McLean. ©2006 Michelle McLean.

Joint Effort. Reprinted by permission of Debra Weaver. ©2006 Debra Weaver.

Dieter's Block. Reprinted by permission of Terry A. Lilley. ©2004 Terry A. Lilley.

Jiggles. Reprinted by permission of Edwina L. Kaikai. ©2001 Edwina L. Kaikai. Portions excerpted from *Stomach in My Lap* (Pneuma Publishing International, Inc., 2004, www.pneumapublishing.com.)

The Exercise Bike. Reprinted by permission of Ann Morrow. ©2004 Ann Morrow.

Weight in the Balance. Reprinted by permission of Laura Schroll. ©2006 Laura Schroll.

Just Listen to Mom. Reprinted by permission of James Hammill. ©2004 James Hammill. Previously published in *Chicken Soup for the Soul Healthy Living, Weight Loss* (Health Communications, Inc., 2004).

Spaghetti Head. Reprinted by permission of Jean Stewart. ©2006 Jean Stewart.

Half My Size. Reprinted by permission of Suzanne Baginskie. ©2006 Suzanne Baginskie.

The Secret. Reprinted by permission of Marilyn Eudaly. ©2004 Marilyn

Eudaly. Previously published in *Chicken Soup for the Soul Healthy Living, Weight Loss* (Health Communcations, Inc., 2004).

Seeing Double. Reprinted by permission of Selena Hayes. ©2006 Selena Hayes.

Drinking Herself Fat. Reprinted by permission of Jennie Ivey. ©2006 Jennie Ivey.

The Un-Diet. Reprinted by permission of Susan A. Karas. ©2006 Susan A. Karas.

It Takes Community. Reprinted by permission of Pamela Wertz Peterson. ©2006 Pamela Wertz Peterson.

In for a Penny, In for a Pound. Reprinted by permission of Ava Pennington. ©2006 Ava Pennington.

The First Day of the Best of My Life. Reprinted by permission of Charmi Schroeder. ©2003 Charmi Schroeder.

Fabulously Fighting Fit at Fifty (and Beyond). Reprinted by permission of Janet Marianne Jackson. ©2005 Janet Marianne Jackson. Originally appeared in *Healthy Options Magazine.*

A Second Chance at Life. Reprinted by permission of Nancy Julien Kopp. ©2002 Nancy Julien Kopp. Previously appeared on www.medhunters.com.

A Soul-Searching, Pound-Shedding Vacation. Reprinted by permission of Jessica Blaire. ©2006 Jessica Blaire.

7 Hints for Navigating Your Supermarket. Reprinted by permission of Tricia Finch. ©2006 Tricia Finch.

Monday Morning Blues. Reprinted by permission of Georgia A. Hubley. ©2004 Georgia A. Hubley. Previously published in *Chicken Soup for the Soul Healthy Living, Weight Loss* (Health Communications, Inc., 2004).

My Last Twenty Pounds. Reprinted by permission of Kate Baggott. ©2005 Kate Baggott.

Setting Goals and Reaping Rewards. Reprinted by permission of Felice Prager. ©2003 Felice Prager.

No More Pancakes on This Woman's Shopping List! Reprinted by permission of Roberta Beach Jacobson. ©2004 Roberta Beach Jacobson. Originally appeared in *Dog & Kennel* (Pet Publishing).

Beating the Genes. Reprinted by permission of Lisa Pemberton. ©2004 Lisa Pemberton.

The Bargain. Reprinted by permission of Delores Christian Liesner. ©2006 Delores Christian Liesner.

Stroke of Inspiration. Reprinted by permission of Charmi Schroeder. ©2006 Charmi Schroeder.

Couch Meets Table. Reprinted by permission of Harriet Cooper. ©2005 Harriet Cooper.

Worship Walk. Reprinted by permission of Jaye Lewis. ©2005 Jaye Lewis.

Resources

We offer the following resources as a service to readers but are not endorsing any of the organizations, programs or books listed.

HEALTH & NUTRITION

American Association of Clinical Endocrinologists

Website: *aace.com*   E-mail: *djones@aace.com*

Provides information to the public about diabetes, thyroid disorders, growth hormone deficiency, osteoporosis, cholesterol disorders, hypertension and obesity.

1000 Riverside Avenue, Suite 205 • Jacksonville, FL 32204
Phone: (904) 353-7878 • Fax: (904) 353-8185

American Diabetes Association

Website: *diabetes.org*   E-mail: *askada@diabetes.org*

Information on all diabetes-related issues.

National Call Center • 1701 N Beauregard Street • Alexandria, VA 22311
Phone: (800) 342-2383

American Dietetic Association

Website: *eatright.org*   E-mail: *foundation@eatright.org*

One of the nation's largest organizations of food and nutrition professionals. Provides a list of dieticians in your area.

120 South Riverside Plaza, Suite 2000 • Chicago, IL 60606
Phone: (800) 877-1600 • Fax: (312) 899-1979

American Heart Association

Website: *americanheart.org*

The source of information for today's health-savvy consumer about low-saturated fat, low-cholesterol alternatives to common high-saturated fat, high-cholesterol food; provides important information on reading food labels and offers tips for raising heart-healthy, active children.

7272 Greenville Avenue • Dallas, TX 75231
Phone: Heart (800) 242-8721 • Phone: Stroke (800) 478-7653

American Obesity Association

Website: *obesity.org*   E-mail: *executive@obesity.org*

One of the most trusted sources for information on obesity. Obesity is associated with insulin resistance, diabetes, hypertension, obstructive sleep apnea, depression, orthopaedic issues and increased risk for serious cardiovascular and liver trouble as well as several types of cancer.

1250 24th Stree NW, Suite 300, • Washington, DC 20037
Phone: (202) 776-7711 • Fax: (202) 776-7712

American Society of Bariatric Physicians

Website: *asbp.org*   E-mail: *info@asbp.org*

Offers information on obesity, tips on weight loss and a referral program to reach member physicians for professional consultation.

2821 South Parker Road, Suite 625 • Aurora, CO 80014
Phone: (303) 770-2526 • Fax: (303) 779-4834

Center for Science in the Public Interest

Website: *cspinet.org*   E-mail: *cspi@cspinet.org*

Advances legislation and promotes healthier food options in restaurants, standards for food labeling and truth in advertising.

1875 Connecticut Avenue NW, Suite 300 • Washington, DC 20009
Phone: (202) 332-9110 • Fax: (202) 265-4954

Chemocare.com, Cleveland Clinic Cancer Center

Website: *chemocare.com*

Diets that you can follow during chemotherapy treatments.

Fitness and Freebies

Website: *fitnessandfreebies.com*

Handy charts for recommended height and weight for adult men and women.

Medilexicon International

Website: *medicalnewstoday.com*

A good source for all news related to health and wellness compiled and updated daily from multiple sources.

Overeater's Anonymous

Website: *oa.org*   E-mail: *info@oa.org*

A program of recovery from compulsive overeating using the Twelve Steps and Twelve Traditions of OA. Worldwide meetings and other tools provide a fellowship of experience, strength and hope where members respect one another's anonymity. OA charges no dues or fees; it is self-supporting through member contributions. It addresses physical, emotional and spiritual well-being. It is not a religious organization and does not promote any particular diet.

World Service Office • P.O. Box 44020 • Rio Rancho, NM 87174
Phone: (505) 891-2664 • Fax: (505) 891-4320

Pregnancy Today

Website: *pregnancytoday.com*

Information on average and recommended weight gain/loss from pregnancy.

United States Department of Agriculture

Website: *mypyramid.gov*   E-mail: *support@cnpp*

A detailed assessment of your food intake and physical activity level that can help you choose the foods and amounts that are right for you. Click on "MyPyramid Tracker." Use the advice to make smart choices from every food group. Find your balance between food and physical activity and get the most nutrition out of your calories.

USDA Center for Nutrition Policy and Promotion
3101 Park Center Drive, Room 1034 • Alexandria, VA 22302

University of Sydney

Website: *glycemicindex.com*

Complete information on the glycemic index, which is a measurement of how fast a food is likely to raise your blood sugar.

WebMD

Website: *webmd.com*

One of the most reliable sources of information on health and wellness on the internet.

Weight Management Resources

Website: *weight-manage.info*

A portal for many weight management sites.

Wellness.com

Website: *wellness.com*

A comprehensive website featuring information on fitness, nutrition and weight management.

Weight-Control Information Network (WIN)

Website: *niddk.nih.gov*   E-mail: *win@info.niddk.nih.gov*

A service of the National Institute of Diabetes and Digestive and Kidney Diseases (NIDDK) that provides the general public, health professionals, the media and Congress with up-to-date, science-based information on weight control, obesity, physical activity and related nutritional issues

1 WIN Way • Bethesda, MD 20892-3665

MENTAL HEALTH & ADVOCACY

Council on Size and Weight Discrimination

Website: *cswd.org*   E-mail: *info@cswd.org*

Provides public education and advocacy on issues of weight discrimination, size acceptance, health at every size and body image issues.

P.O. Box 305 • Mount Marion, NY 12456
Phone: (845) 679-1209 • Fax: (845) 679-1206

National Eating Disorders Association

Website: *edap.org*   E-mail: *info@NationalEatingDisorders.org*

The National Eating Disorders Association (NEDA) is the largest not-for-profit organization in the United States working to prevent eating disorders and provide treatment referrals to those suffering from anorexia, bulimia and binge eating disorder, and body image and weight issues.

603 Stewart Street, Suite 803 • Seattle, WA 98101
Phone: (800) 931-2237

FITNESS

American Council on Exercise

Website: *acefitness.org*   E-mail: *resource@acefitness.org*

The largest nonprofit fitness certification and education provider in the world. Sets standards and protects the public against unqualified fitness professionals and unsafe or ineffective fitness products, programs and trends.

4851 Paramount Drive • San Diego, CA 92123
Phone: (800) 825-3636 • Fax: (858) 279-8064

American Running Association

Website: *americanrunning.org*   E-mail: *run@americanrunning.org*

Information and support for runners from runners and medical professionals.

4405 East West Hwy, Suite 405 • Bethesda, MD 20814
Phone: (800) 776-2732 • Fax: (301) 913 9520

Aquatic Exercise Association

Website: *aeawave.com*   E-mail: *info@aeawave.com*

Information on health and fitness through aquatic exercise.

201 Tamiami Trail South, Suite 3 • Nokomis, FL 34275
Phone: (941) 486-8600 • Fax: (941) 486-8820

Boston University Nutrition & Fitness Center

Website: *bu.edu/nfc*   E-mail: *nfc@bu.edu*

Individual and group nutrition and fitness programs, as well as health screenings, fitness evaluations and workshops.

635 Commonwealth Avenue, Room 401 • Boston, MA 02215
Phone: (617) 353-2721

Global Health & Fitness

Website: *global-fitness.com*   E-mail: *info@global-fitness.com*

Online membership-based program that teaches you how to implement all five components of fitness: strength training, weight management, cardiovascular exercise, nutrition and flexibility training in combinations that recognize your goals and are realistic for your level of experience and for the time you can commit.

P.O. Box 2696 • Clackamas, OR 97015
Phone: (503) 772-4299

PLANS & PROGRAMS

Atkins

Website: *atkins.com*

The Atkins diet allows for up to two-thirds of calories to come from fat, more than twice usual recommendations. Atkins emphasizes meat, eggs and cheese. It discourages bread, rice and fruit. Weight loss is often sustained and followers see a marked improvement in their triglyceride levels and a loss in body fat.

eDiets

Website: *ediet.com* E-mail: *help@ediets.com*

A web-based membership program that offers twenty-four personalized online programs featuring all the popular diet plans and ten proprietary programs for those with special needs. Members choose a plan and complete a personal profile to determine how to best custom-tailor the program for their unique needs. Members have 24/7/365 access to *eDiets.com*'s community for motivation and support from *eDiets.com*'s on-staff experts and member peers.

1000 Corporate Drive, Suite 600 • Ft Lauderdale, FL 33334
Phone: (800) 265-6170 • Fax: (954) 360-9095

Jenny Craig

Website: *jennycraig.com*

A three-level, food/mind/body plan. At the first level, the program teaches clients how to eat the foods they want in small, frequent portions. At the second level, the program teaches clients how to increase their energy levels via simple activity. At the third level, the program addresses building more balance into clients' lives in order to maintain weight loss and healthy diet. The program offers several levels of support, including a 24/7 telephone line.

Perricone Program

Website: *nvperriconemd.com*

Dr. Nicholas V. Perricone, a world-renowned dermatologist, concluded that inflammation significantly contributes to aging, weight gain, fatigue, disease and skin problems. He developed an anti-aging and anti-inflammatory diet for his skin-care patients that reduces damage caused by free radicals to the outer layer of cells. It stresses nutrition and supplementation by eating a diet of fish, low-glycemic index foods, olive oil, fruits and vegetables, and omega 3, 6 and 9 fatty acids.

N.V. Perricone, M.D., Ltd. • 639 Research Parkway • Meriden, CT 06450
Phone: (888) 823-7837 • Fax: (203) 379-0817

South Beach Diet

Website: *southbeachdiet.com*

The key elements of the South Beach Diet are good fats like olive and canola oil, the omega-3 fish oils, and oils found in most nuts combined with good carbohydrates, which are vegetables, whole-grain breads and whole fruits. Strategic snacking is encouraged to keep hunger under control and prevent cravings. Attention is paid to the glycemic index, which is a measure of how quickly a carbohydrate raises your blood sugar.

The Mediterranean Diet

Website: *medidiet/rescources.com*

The classic Mediterranean diet recommended by the American Heart Association consists of high consumption of fruits, vegetables, bread and other cereals, potatoes, beans, nuts and seeds. Olive oil is an important mono-unsaturated fat source. Dairy products, fish and poultry are consumed in low to moderate amounts, and little red meat is eaten. Eggs are consumed no more than four times a week. Wine is consumed in low to moderate amounts. People who follow the average Mediterranean diet eat less saturated fat than those who eat the average American diet.

The Schwarzbein Principle

Website: *schwarzbeinprinciple.com*   E-mail: *info@schwarzbeinprinciple.com*

Diana Schwarzbein, an endocrinologist and internist, concluded that by cutting carbohydrates and adding proteins and fats, most type 2 diabetes patients started losing one to two pounds of body fat per week (after initial body-water loss). Patients following her program have seen their blood sugars normalize, cholesterol levels improve, blood pressures come down, and a loss of body fat and gain in muscle mass.

5901 Encina Road, Suite A • Goleta, CA 93117

The Zone

Website: *zonediet.com*

Zone Diet meals follow the hand-eye method. One-third of your plate consists of a serving of lean protein no bigger than the size and thickness of the palm of your hand. The other two-thirds is filled with favorable carbohydrates, such as fruits and vegetables. Finally, a dash of "good" fat, such as nuts, olive oil or avocado, is added. You eat three meals a day, plus two snacks, and never go more than five hours without eating, so you don't feel deprived.

Tops Club Inc.

Website: *tops.org*

Founded in 1948, TOPS (Take Off Pounds Sensibly) is the oldest international, nonprofit, noncommercial weight-loss support group. TOPS program components provide weekly meetings, include private weigh-ins, and provides members with positive reinforcement and motivation to adhere to food and exercise plans. Since 1966, TOPS has funded an obesity and metabolic research program at the Medical College of Wisconsin in Milwaukee and supports ongoing research there. To date, $5.4 million from TOPS earnings and member contributions have helped fund obesity research.

Weight Watchers

Website: *weightwatchers.com*

Combining weekly meetings and a healthy food plan with behavioral modification and exercise, Weight Watchers is one of the most popular weight management programs in the world. The Weight Watcher "points" system, allows you to enjoy any food you like as long as you control how much you eat. They also offer a "core plan" that focuses on eating foods from all the food groups, even an occasional treat. Members get weighed in weekly and soak up the support from fellow dieters. Meetings are held in thousands of cities around the world, and Weight Watchers low-calorie, portion-controlled foods are readily available in most supermarkets. Members get exercise tips, recipes, the benefits of scientific research, and ongoing motivational coaching and support.

The Diet Channel

Website: *thedietchannel.com*

TheDietChannel.com is an award-winning health, nutrition and weight loss resource. Founded in the mid-90s it features links and reviews of today's popular diet programs as well as in-depth articles by contributing writers who are experts in the field. *TheDietChannel.com* also maintains an index of some of the best nutrition sites on the Internet.

TREATMENT & RESEARCH

Massachusetts General Hospital Weight Center

Website: *massgeneral.org/weightc*   E-mail: *weightcenter@partners.org*

Expert consultation and treatment for both adults and children, emphasizing family-based therapy whenever appropriate. Offers a complete range of services to overweight patients, from nutritional, exercise and psychological counseling to state-of-the-art medical and surgical treatment of weight disorders. Life-long care of patients and programs are offered to encourage close, long-term follow-up.

50 Staniford Street, 4th Floor • Boston, MA 02114
Phone: (617) 726-4400 • Fax: (617) 724-6565

University of Alabama at Birmingham
EatRight Weight Management Program

Website: *main.uab.edu/sites/eatright*   E-mail: *strongdc@uab.edu*

EatRight is a lifestyle-oriented weight control program designed to beat the odds of the weight-loss battle by easing participants into new eating and exercising habits. Based on the findings that the amount of food we eat, rather than the caloric or the fat content of the food, determines when we feel full and stop eating. The expert team of physicians, dietitians and exercise trainers provides EatRight services to the general public using the most up-to-date nutrition information available.

AB 1064 • 1530 3rd Avenue, South • Birmingham, AL 35294
Phone: (205) 934-7053

St. Luke's-Hospital Center VanItallie Center for Nutrition and Weight Management

Website: *uchsc.edu/core/newyork.htm*

A program for weight loss for the short term and weight maintenance for the long term. Weekly, all patients have their blood pressure checked and are given the opportunity to speak with a clinical assistant, nurse or dietitian. Each patient also participates in a weekly group class and sees the physician no less than monthly. Treatments for weight loss are effective but purposefully do not result in rapid weight loss. Whether weight loss is accomplished with the help of liquid formula, regular food, surgery or medication, staff monitor patients to ensure that they lose as much fat as possible, but not at the expense of lean tissue such as skeletal muscle, the heart, the liver and the skin. Also holds workshops on topics such as low-fat cooking, exercise and stress reduction to promote better health and nutrition.

425 West 59th Street, #9D • New York, NY 10019
Phone: (212) 523-8440

The New York Obesity Research Center Weight Loss Program

Website: *nyorc.org/weightlossprogram*　　　E-mail: *dg108@columbia.edu*

Groups meet once a week for one year and are led by highly skilled and experienced professionals, ready with the newest and most effective strategies to help clients lose weight and keep it off.

1090 Amsterdam Avenue, 14th Floor • New York, NY 10025
Phone: (212) 523-8440 • Fax: (212) 523-3416

University of Colorado Center for Human Nutrition

Website: *uchsc.edu/nutrition*

Research conducted at the CHN focuses on obesity prevention and treatment, nutrient metabolism, and micronutrient status in children. The community outreach activities initiated and conducted through the CHN aim to improve quality of life by promoting physical activity and nutritional awareness.

Campus Box C290 • 4200 East Ninth Avenue • Denver, CO 80262
Phone: (303) 372-0000

Duke University Diet and Fitness Center

Website: *cfl.duke.edu*　　　E-mail: *dfcinfo@dukedietcenter.org*

The Center's staff is skilled in weight management, but also guides patients to substantially increase physical activity, which is as equally important as eating healthfully. Clients learn strategies conducive to weight management while maximizing overall health. Goals are to reduce the risk of heart disease and cancer, to minimize disability from arthritis and chronic pain and to build stamina, mobility and lung function, while managing stress and improving mood. This program is not for everyone. It requires a significant investment in time, money and energy. Those who have not given serious attention to less intensive approaches should perhaps try those first. This is a place for folks who are serious about charting a new path to better health.

804 West Trinity Avenue • Durham, NC 27701
Phone: (800) 235-3853 • Fax: (919) 684-8246

Loma Linda University Center for Health Promotion

Website: *llu.edu/llu/chp*

A free, informative one-hour session designed to describe the various weight management programs and helps clients decide what program will best meet their needs. The Optifast program is a twenty-six week, medically supervised program for individuals with fifty or more pounds to lose. Lean Choices is a twelve-week class for those who want to improve their health and weight through exercise, food choices and the psychology of eating.

Evans Hall • 24785 Stewart Street • Loma Linda, CA 92350
Phone: (909) 558-4594

Scripps Clinic Nutrition and Metabolic Research Center

Website: *scrippshealth.org*

A comprehensive program for adults, adolescents and pediatrics covering every aspect of weight management for both underweight patients and those struggling with morbid obesity. Includes clinical trials testing everything from hormones, diets and medical devices to supplements, herbal preparations and nutritional aids. Also provides a full complement of care for types 1 and 2 diabetes (pediatric and adult), thyroid disease, pediatric growth and development, osteoporosis, and pituitary and adrenal disorders. Medically supervised, individualized exercise, nutritional and psychological programs are available. Specialists study the genetic abnormalities of obesity to accurately diagnose the cause of weight gain and plan for its care.

12395 El Camino Real, Suite 317 • San Diego, CA 92130
Phone: (866) 444-3638 • Fax: (858) 794-1244

University of Cincinnati Obesity Research Center

Website: *psychiatry.uc.edu/orc*

Conducts basic scientific research on the regulation of body weight and the etiology and potential treatment of obesity. It encompasses several laboratories from various departments at the University of Cincinnati College of Medicine.

Dept of Psychiatry • Genome Research Institute
2170 East Galbraith Road • Bldg. E Room 308 • Cincinnati, OH 45237
Phone: (513) 558-6863 • Fax: (513) 558-8990

University of Pittsburgh Obesity/Nutrition Research Center

Website: *pitt.edu/~onrc*   E-mail: *casiled@dom.pitt.edu*

Focuses on behavioral aspects of obesity and behavioral treatment of obesity. A patient-oriented research facility. Assessing the impact of current treatments of obesity is a key part of their focus. These assessments include examining metabolic and genetic factors related to insulin resistance, the impact of obesity and other nutrition-related illnesses on body composition, and examining behavioral, pharmacological and surgical treatments of obesity.

200 Lothrop Street • Pittsburgh, PA 15213-2582
Phone: 1-800-533-UPMC (8762)

Yale Center for Eating and Weight Disorders

Website: *yale.edu/ycewd*   E-mail: *ycewd@yale.edu*

Provides services to members of the community to better understand eating and weight disorders.

P.O. Box 208205 • New Haven, CT 06520
Phone: (203) 432-4610

BOOKS

Body Image

Do I Look Fat in This? Get Over Your Body and On with Your Life
Rhonda Britten

Women befriend their bodies—first by facing and accepting what they see in the mirror, and then by empowering them to make healthier decisions about their weight.

ISBN 0525949453 • 272 pages • hardcover • $24.95 • Penguin Group • 2006

Intuitive Eating: A Revolutionary Program That Works
Evelyn Tribole, M.S., R.D., Elyse Resch, M.S., R.D., F.A.D.A.

Two prominent nutritionists focus on nurturing your body rather than starving it. Encourages natural weight loss and helps you find the weight you were meant to be. Compassionate, thoughtful advice on satisfying, healthy living

ISBN 0312321236 • 304 pages • paperback • $13.95 • St. Martin's Press • 2003

Life Without Ed: How One Woman Declared Independence from Her Eating Disorder and How You Can Too

Jenni Schaefer

Eight million women in the United States suffer from anorexia nervosa and/or bulimia. For these women, the road to recovery is a rocky one where many succumb to their eating disorders. Readers are encouraged to think of an eating disorder as if it were a distinct being with a personality of its own. Further, they are encouraged to treat the disorder as a relationship rather than as a condition.

ISBN 0071422986 • 192 pages • paperback • $14.95 • McGraw-Hill • 2003

Children's Obesity/Weight Management

Ending the Food Fight, Guide Your Child to a Healthy Weight in a Fast Food/Fake Food World

David S. Ludwig, M.D., Ph.D., with Suzanne Rostler, M.S., R.D.

High-calorie, low-quality fast food and "fake food" (processed foods unlike anything found in nature), present a serious challenge for parents managing their children's weight. Harvard endocrinologist Dr. David Ludwig's groundbreaking research in the use of a low-glycemic diet to combat obesity is the basis for some of the most successful diets of the last decade. Dr. Ludwig's low-glycemic diet combined with a powerful, nine-week progressive plan addresses biology, behavior and environment and integrates them into a practical prescription for weight loss. Dr. Ludwig gives parents all the tools they need to help their children win the food fight once and for all.

ISBN 0618683267 • 320 pages • hardcover • $26.00
Houghton-Mifflin • April 2007

Diet Plans

American Heart Association No-Fad Diet:
A Personal Plan for Healthy Weight Loss

After a simple assessment of your current habits, you choose the eating and exercise strategies that best fit your needs. You'll learn how to set realistic goals, eat well to lose extra pounds safely and add physical activity to keep the weight off for good. This book offers more than 190 delicious, all-new recipes, two weeks of sample menus, guidelines for meal planning, useful tips on dining out and food shopping, and sound advice for staying on track to reach your target weight.

ISBN 1400051592 • 464 pages • hardcover • $24.95 • Clarkson Potter • 2005

Dr. Gott's No Flour, No Sugar Diet
Peter H. Gott, M.D.

A sensible guide for healthy eating that will help you achieve your desired weight and maintain it for life. Simple, inexpensive, easy to follow, nutritious, and easy to maintain over the long haul. Eliminate flour and added sugar from your diet. You'll still enjoy lean meats, brown rice, low-fat dairy products, vegetables, fruits and other goodies. Allows foods from all the food groups, so you'll be getting all the nutrients you need to maintain a healthy body while shedding unwanted pounds.

ISBN 1884956521 • 244 pages • paperback • $14.95
Quill Driver Books • 2006

How to Make Almost Any Diet Work
Anne Katherine

Bestselling author and psychotherapist Anne Katherine—herself a recovering overeater—specializes in treating appetite disorders and food addictions. Discusses the chemistry behind appetite, hunger, fullness and satiety and gives focused activities to decrease appetite and increase satiety. Working from the premise that most overeaters use food as a comfort drug, the reader learns how to acquire comfort from other, healthier sources. Provides practical tools to help the reader analyze his/her own body chemistry to choose the diet that will best fit his/her needs.

ISBN 1592853579 • 250 pages • paperback • $14.95 • Hazelden • 2006

The 90/10 Weight-Loss Plan
Joy Bauer, M.S., R.D., C.D.N.

The 90/10 plan provides approximately 50 percent of total calories from quality carbohydrates, moderate amounts from lean protein and limited amounts from fat—proportions that research has proven to be optimal for good health and disease prevention. The meal plans are balanced to provide you with the most vitamins and minerals possible for the controlled amount of calories consumed. Menus are also low in saturated fat and dietary cholesterol, and high in fiber, phytochemicals and antioxidants.

ISBN 0312303971 • 304 pages • paperback • $13.95
St Martin's Griffin • 2002

The Cheater's Diet: The Medically Proven Way to Supercharge Your Weight Loss, Break Through Diet Ruts and Stay Thin for Good
Paul Rivas, M.D., and Ernie Tremblay

From helping over 15,000 people lose weight, Dr. Paul Rivas discovered people who cheat on their diets lose weight the fastest and keep it off the longest. He explains this scientifically validated secret that ends yo-yo dieting: It's not whether you cheat on your diet (because you will!), but how and when you do it. He not only encourages you, but requires you to indulge in delicious foods such as chocolate, wine, cinnamon buns, beer and pizza. The healthiest, most effective weekday eating plan known to science with doctor-approved recipes that are simple and delicious

ISBN 0757303218 • 203 pages • hardcover • $18.95

Health Communications, Inc. • 2005

The DASH Diet Action Plan

Marla Heller, M.S., R.D.

The 2005 dietary guidelines for Americans recommends this eating plan for everyone, and the DASH diet forms the basis for the new MyPyramid. The diet is rich in fruits, vegetables, low-fat or nonfat dairy, and includes lean meats, fish and poultry, grains, nuts and beans. It helps lower cholesterol and supports healthy weight loss. This book is designed to make it easy to put the DASH program into practice in your life, showing how to eat on-the-run, how to add more vegetables even if you hate vegetables, how to make over your kitchen to support the DASH diet, and how to lose weight with the DASH diet.

ISBN 0976340801 • 223 pages • paperback • $19.95 • Amidon Press • 2005

The Fat Smash Diet

Ian K. Smith, M.D.

Not a gimmick or short-term fix. It is a four-phase diet that starts out with a natural detox phase to clean impurities out of the system. Once this nine-day phase is completed, the next three phases encourage the addition of everyday foods that promote significant weight loss. In just thirty days, most dieters will complete all four phases. There is no calorie counting, and as an added bonus, there are over fifty easy-to-cook, tasty recipes that make it easier to stick with the plan.

ISBN 0312363133 • 159 pages • paperback • $12.95 • St. Martin's Press • 2006

The Rice Diet Solution

Kitty Gurkin Rosati, M.S., R.D., L.D.N., and Robert Roseti, M.D.

Men lose on average twenty-eight to thirty pounds and women on average nineteen to twenty pounds per month on this diet! The Rice Diet also detoxes your body, ridding it of excess water weight and toxins from processed foods and the environment. The program's results have been documented by extensive studies and confirmed by thousands of people who report amazing weight loss, as well as immediate improvement in such conditions as heart disease, diabetes and hypertension. Includes hundreds of tasty, filling, easy-to-prepare recipes—some from the Rice

House kitchen, others inspired by major chefs and adapted to Rice Diet standards. Not just an eating plan, but a physical, emotional and spiritual program that will give you new vitality, energy and longevity.
ISBN 0743289838 • 368 pages • hardcover • $25.00
Simon & Schuster • 2005

You: On a Diet: The Owner's Manual for Waist Management
Michael F. Roizen, M.D., and Mehmet C. Oz, M.D.
A wealth of material that tests your weight-management IQ and busts popular myths about dieting and weight loss. The diet and exercise plans are easy to follow and the authors discuss medical intervention, drugs and surgery.
ISBN 0743292545 • 384 pages • hardcover • $25.00 • Free Press • 2006

Health & Fitness

DietMinder: Personal Food & Fitness Journal: A Deluxe Food Diary
MemoryMinder Journals
The roomy, fill-in-the-blank format gives you plenty of space for the detailed entries. It's organized and easy to use. The Goals section sets you on a clear and defined plan of action. The Daily Record pages guide you effortlessly through breakfast, lunch, dinner, snacks, supplements and daily exercise. Totaling your food counts and using the Progress Charts is a breeze! Other sections include basic Guidelines for daily servings, nutritional recommendations and a "calories burned" chart. The handy Favorite Foods section includes food count information on over 100 common foods and can be customized by adding your own favorites.
ISBN 0963796836 • 224 pages • spiral • $14.95
MemoryMinder Journals • 2000

The Gold Coast Cure: The 5-Week Health and Body Makeover
Andrew Larson, M.D. and Ivy Ingram Larson
Multiple sclerosis left Ivy Larson wearing a catheter and unable to walk up a flight of stairs at the age of twenty-two. Undeterred, she and her husband, Dr. Andrew Larson, devised an anti-inflammatory whole foods diet and exercise plan to heal her. It worked. Today, her MS is in remission and she has the extra energy to keep up with their healthy toddler. The plan has helped people reverse obesity, coronary artery disesase, type 2 diabetes, multiple sclerosis, asthma, allergies, osteoarthritis, fibromyalgia, osteoporosis and vascular dementia.
ISBN 0757305636, 300 pages, paperback, $15.95
Health Communications, 2007

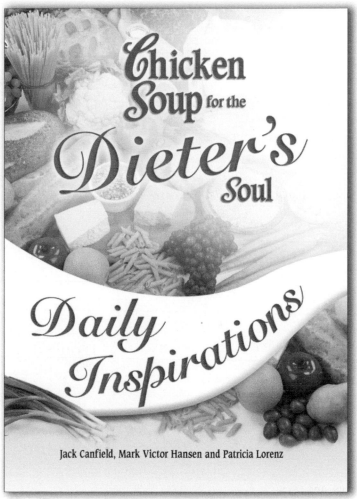

Chicken Soup for the Dieter's Soul

Daily Inspirations

Jack Canfield, Mark Victor Hansen and Patricia Lorenz

Code #5261 • paperback • $14.95

Get the must-have companion
book for any weight-loss program.

To order direct:
Telephone (800) 441-5569 • www.hcibooks.com
Prices do not include shipping and handling. Your response code is CCS.

The Gold Coast Cure's Fitter, Firmer, Faster Program, A 5-Week Total Body Transformation Plan without Going to Extremes

Andrew Larson, M.D., and Ivy Ingram Larson

This high-calorie eating plan allows you to lose weight and prevent disease. It includes brand-name shopping lists, delicious no-fuss recipes, meal plans and a circuit training workout that burns three times more fat than aerobics in just three workouts a week.

ISBN 0757305563 • 268 pages • paperback • $15.95
Health Communications • 2006

The Schwarzbein Principle II: The Transition

Diana Schwarzbein, M.D.

A groundbreaking follow-up look at how your current health is being compromised with a 5-step "transition" plan to heal your metabolism.

ISBN 1558749640 • 380 pages • paperback • $14.95
Health Communications • 2002

The Schwarzbein Principle Cookbook

Diana Schwarzbein, M.D., Nancy Deville and Evelyn Jacob Jaffe

From the Schwarzbein Institute come 300 delicious, healing recipes with easy-to-follow directions, tips and comprehensive nutritional breakdowns.

ISBN 1558746811 • 380 pages • paperback • $12.95
Health Communications • 1999

You, the Owner's Manual: An Insider's Guide to the Body That Will Make You Healthier and Younger

Michael F. Roizen, M.D. and Mehmet C. Oz, M.D.

Instead of dry, impenetrable scientific jargon, Doctors Mehmet Oz and Michael Roizen describe each integral part of the body (including organs, bones, and immune system) in terms that readers can understand and use. This is a health book like no other.

ISBN 0060765313 • 417 pages • hardcover • $24.95 • HarperCollins • 2005